SO-AWB-232

Developmental Problems of Drug-Exposed Infants

Edited by

Louis M. Rossetti, Ph.D.

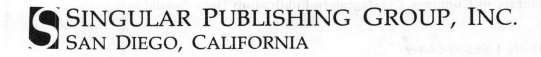

SINGULAR PUBLISHING GROUP, INC.
SAN DIEGO, CALIFORNIA

Singular Publishing Group, Inc.
4284 41st Street
San Diego, California 92105-1197

© **1992 by Singular Publishing Group, Inc.**

Typeset in 10/12 Souvenir by CFW Graphics
Printed in the United States of America by McNaughton & Gunn

All rights, including that of translation, reserved. No part of this publication may be reproduced, stored in a retrieval system, or transmitted in any form or by any means, electronic, mechanical, recording, or otherwise, without the prior written permission of the publisher.

Library of Congress Cataloging-in-Publication Data Available

ISBN 1-56593-064-9

Contents

Preface

Since 1985 the number of children prenatally exposed to drugs has tripled. In 1989 the number of drug-exposed infants and toddlers in the United States comprised 11% of all live births. Clearly, the demand for services for this unique population of infants, toddlers, and their families far exceeds the availability of trained personnel. Clinicians from various disciplines report that providing early intervention services for drug-exposed infants and toddlers presents them with unique challenges. In addition, working with caregivers, who must be included in early intervention activities, is equally challenging.

This book is designed to provide clinically relevant information on drug-exposed infants to early interventionists. The authors represent medicine, speech-language pathology, early childhood special education, audiology, social work, and developmental psychology. Issues relative to working with families, medical concerns, language characteristics, behavioral characteristics, audiological concerns, and the impact on schools are addressed.

It is anticipated that this book will become an important addition to your professional library — one that you can refer to often and that you can recommend to colleagues interested in a transdisciplinary approach toward providing effective services to drug-exposed infants, toddlers, and their families. Each of the authors is clinically active in service provision to drug-exposed infants. I know that you will find their insights helpful and challenging.

Developmental Problems of Drug-Exposed Infants has been published in book form simultaneously with its release as Volume 2, Number 1 of *Infant-Toddler Intervention: The Transdisciplinary Journal.* Published information on this fast-breaking topic has been sparse while the need for it has been in great demand. We have released this book especially for professionals who *must* have reliable, up-to-date information on drug-exposed infants.

Acknowledgments

I would like to acknowledge the editorial assistance provided by Ruth Stonestreet and Mark Heffner who reviewed the articles by Sharon Lesar and Charles MacDonald, respectively. Additional editorial reviews on all other articles were provided by Margaret H. Briggs, Jack Kile, Sharon Raver-Lampman, Charles MacDonald, Anna Simpson, Joan Sogard, Joyce W. Sparling, and Melanie Spence.

Perinatal Cocaine Exposure: Predictor of an Endangered Generation

Charles C. MacDonald, M.D.

Special Care Nursery
St. Mary's Medical Center
Evansville, Indiana

The increased frequency of maternal cocaine abuse during pregnancy has caused a tremendous clinical impact on the immediate and long-term care of infants exposed to the drug during gestation. Estimates of the number of women abusing cocaine at any time during pregnancy range from 11 to 25%. The use of the drug crosses all social, economic, and racial lines. Intensive care nurseries are becoming overburdened with the immediate medical problems of cocaine-exposed babies; foster care systems are overwhelmed with abandoned and/or medically high-risk infants; and the school systems predict great difficulties in providing for the educational needs of this potentially large group of high-risk children.

Cocaine is one of a group of commonly abused drugs that easily crosses the placental barrier and upon reaching the fetus may create hazards for fetal development. Cocaine has been associated with prematurity, intrauterine growth retardation, congenital anomalies, and long-term neurodevelopmental deficits. Its inherent ability to disrupt the maternal-fetal vascular system in addition to having probable direct cellular biochemical effects allows cocaine to affect the fetus at any stage of development.

This article addresses the problems involved in recognition of maternal chemical abuse, the pharmacologic effects of cocaine on the pregnant mother and her fetus, and the ramifications of prenatal cocaine abuse on medical, legal, and social issues.

Epidemiology of Cocaine Abuse in Pregnancy

Since the early 1970s when fetal alcohol syndrome was first described, maternal abuse of chemical substances during pregnancy has escalated to the point where large numbers of infants are being admitted to intensive care nurseries for treatment of complications from intrauterine exposure to illicit drugs.

In 1988, 11% of all women delivering at 36 hospitals surveyed in the United States had ingested one, or more, illegal drugs dur-

Infant-Toddler Intervention.
The Transdisciplinary Journal (Vol. 2, No. 1, pp. 1–12)
© 1992, Singular Publishing Group, Inc.

ing pregnancy (Chasnoff, 1989). Several other large studies have been completed since then, confirming that 11 to 25% of pregnant women abuse chemical substances during pregnancy. In a population-based study of 715 pregnant women entering the health care system during a 6-month period in Pinellas County, Florida, 15% of the women had a positive urine screen for cocaine, marijuana, or heroin (Chasnoff, Landress, & Barrett, 1990). Further examination of the women revealed no differences in rates of positive screens between the public and private sectors. This study makes it clear that illicit drug use during pregnancy crosses all racial, ethnic, and socioeconomic boundaries.

The difficulties in performing accurate studies on the number of pregnant women abusing drugs revolve around the methodology used to ascertain substance abuse. It is difficult in many studies to obtain reliable historical information from mothers because of the current social and legislative attitude toward pregnant substance abusers — mothers using illegal drugs during pregnancy are unlikely to divulge that information in fear of legal retribution. Indeed, in many states, evidence of chemical abuse during pregnancy is considered child abuse and action to have the infant taken away from the mother may occur after birth. Urine toxicology screens are dependent on the time of ingestion of the drug in relation to when the urine sample is obtained. Detection of illegal substances in the urine of the newborn is also dependent on when the last dose was administered prior to delivery. Newer methodologies, including neonatal meconium screening and maternal/newborn hair analysis, are becoming more accurate in the diagnosis of long-term chemical exposure, but they remain time consuming and expensive to perform.

Chasnoff (1991, p. 117) stated "The cocaine abusing population is a chaotic one,

prone to abrupt changes in lifestyle and drug use patterns." It is common for substance-abusing mothers to be using more than one drug at a time. Cocaine use frequently is accompanied by the use of alcohol, marijuana, and heroin. The drugs may be used in any combination, or over any time periods. These drugs all exert different effects on the fetus and newborn, making large-scale studies of cocaine-only exposed infants difficult to perform and analyze.

Studies by Madden, Payne, and Miller (1986) and Hume et al. (1989) identified populations of women as cocaine abusers, but did not investigate the possibility of polydrug abuse. Little et al. (1989) identified polydrug abuse in their study of cocaine-abusing pregnant women, but did not utilize the data to determine effects of multiple drugs on the eventual outcome of the pregnancies. The population of women abusing cocaine and other types of chemical substances at different stages of pregnancy, in varying combinations, amounts, and frequencies is so diverse that tremendous obstacles are created in statistically analyzing the effects of the drugs, cocaine in particular, on the fetus and infant.

The determination of the stage of pregnancy when a mother uses cocaine and/or other drugs may also affect the results of outcome studies. Chouteau, Numerow, and Leppert (1988) utilized a single urine toxicology screen obtained at the time of delivery to identify mothers using cocaine. However, one negative drug screen does not guarantee drug-free status of the mother throughout pregnancy. Chasnoff et al. (1985) prenatally identified a group of women at risk for cocaine abuse and followed the patterns of their drug use throughout pregnancy. This follow-up allowed more accurate determination of the pattern and timing of cocaine abuse in this population but could not account for the quantity and quality of cocaine ingested, which made it difficult to determine a dose-effect relationship for pregnancy complications secondary to cocaine abuse.

Studies of cocaine-abusing women are also complicated by the various forms of using the drug: inhaled, smoked, free-based, or injected. Different routes of administration of cocaine lead to different blood level concentrations and dose-effect relationships. The quality and concentration of the cocaine may vary over the period of gestation, making comparative studies even more difficult.

Determining the effect of cocaine on a pregnant woman and her fetus requires comparing a population of these women to a socially, biologically, and environmentally similar group of pregnant women who are not abusing cocaine, or other chemical substances, to control for all the independent variables that might adversely affect the pregnancy outcome. Maternal medical histories, frequencies of low birth weight infants, frequencies of congenital malformations to maternal age, race, and socioeconomic background must all be accounted and controlled for, so that cocaine is not spuriously blamed for an adverse pregnancy outcome. Pregnant women may differ genetically in their ability to metabolize and excrete cocaine. The developing fetus also may exhibit different degrees of genetic susceptibility to the drug when compared to another fetus — another factor complicating research on effects and outcomes of cocaine-associated pregnancies.

The many variables involved in developing a longitudinal, controlled study of cocaine abuse during pregnancy make long-term predictions of pregnancy outcome difficult and, at times, erroneous. However, the difficulties involved do not alleviate the need to continue to develop more complex, prospective, comparative studies to further identify the risks associated with prenatal cocaine abuse to the pregnant woman and her child.

Effects of Cocaine on the Pregnant Mother, Fetus, and Newborn

Cocaine is a rapidly acting cerebrocortical stimulant extracted from the leaves of the coca bush and used in South America for hundreds of years to reduce fatigue and induce a state of euphoria. It is imported illegally into the United States and used in several forms and methods. As a powder it may be inhaled nasally ("snorting"); in a volatilized form it may be smoked ("crack"); or it may be injected intravenously, alone, or in combination with other substances (heroin, methadone, and so on).

The route of administration and the form in which cocaine is ingested are variables that complicate the research on its effects on the pregnant mother and fetus. Inhaled in its smoke form, cocaine rapidly diffuses across the lungs into the systemic circulation, achieving a high blood level followed by rapid metabolism and clearance. The euphoric state is achieved to a greater degree and with more rapidity than "snorting" the powder. Intranasal administration results in a slower uptake and delayed clearance because of the local vasoconstriction cocaine causes in the nasal mucosa. This produces a prolonged exposure to the drug but requires a smaller dose. Those women smoking "crack" or injecting the drug intravenously need to administer higher doses to achieve the desired effect and may subsequently experience more toxicity.

Animal and human studies have shown that cocaine may produce complex direct and indirect effects on the maternal-fetal cardiovascular systems in addition to direct effects on the peripheral vascular systems. Cocaine easily crosses the placental barrier reaching significant blood levels rapidly in the developing fetus. Studies by Woods et al. (1989) show a dose-related response between the concentration of intravenously administered cocaine, decreased placental blood flow, increased uterine vascular resistance, increased fetal heart rate, and decreased fetal oxygen content. Although it is difficult to separate the prenatal effect of cocaine from that of multiple drug exposure, there is mounting evidence that cocaine itself during pregnancy is associated with recognizable patterns of adverse outcomes, the majority of which are secondary to decreased fetal, uterine, and placental blood flow. Table 1 describes the most consistently associated abnormalities resulting from prenatal cocaine abuse. Chasnoff et al. (1985) reported placental abnormalities predisposing to placental abruption in 60% of 20 pregnant cocaine users. Chasnoff and Griffith (1989) reported an increased incidence of abruptio placenta (premature separation of the placenta from the uterine wall) and premature delivery in mothers who abused cocaine prenatally. It has been suggested, based on this study and several similar studies, that the hypertensive and

Table 1. Clinical Features Associated with Prenatal Cocaine Abuse

Placental abruption
Prematurity
Intrauterine growth retardation
Central nervous system hemorrhage/infarction
Developmental-behavioral problems
Intestinal obstruction-infarction
Necrotizing enterocolitis
Limb reduction deficits
Urinary tract abnormalities
Myocardial infarction

vasoconstrictive effects of cocaine are most likely responsible for these findings.

The phenomena of intrauterine growth retardation has been well documented in cocaine-abusing mothers and is most likely due to the reduction in placental blood flow and increased uterine vascular resistance. This combination of events decreases the amount of blood flow to the developing fetus, thereby decreasing necessary nutrients and oxygen. The lifestyles of these mothers alone could also affect fetal growth, regardless of the use of drugs. Animal studies demonstrating fetal growth retardation secondary to cocaine have not been conclusive, because the dose necessary to cause adverse fetal effects in the animals studied has been toxic to the mothers. Experimental models to elaborate upon the effect of cocaine on fetal growth need to be developed.

The effects of cocaine abuse on the developing central nervous system (CNS) of the fetus are the most disturbing. Animal studies indicate that cocaine may indirectly alter neurobiochemical function. It has been found by using dopamine-specific ligands in animals that cocaine exposure during pregnancy altered central nervous system dopaminergic function, although similar studies have not been performed in humans. Kramer et al. (1990) speculated that neonatal seizures in cocaine-exposed infants without obvious structural changes in brain anatomy may be secondary to transient changes in neurochemistry and may be precursors of long-term CNS changes and epilepsy. Doberczak et al. (1988) studied 39 infants exposed to cocaine prenatally. Thirty-four (87%) were found to have central nervous system irritability on physical examination and 17 (43%) had abnormal electroencephalograms (EEG) showing cerebral irritation with bursts of sharp waves and spikes in the first week of life. Although no clinical seizures were recognized in this group of infants, the EEG findings remained abnormal for the first 3 to 12 months.

The direct effects of cocaine on the developing fetal brain have been well documented in animals and human infants. Chasnoff et al. (1986) were among the first to suggest that the patterns of intracerebral hemorrhage and cerebral infarction noted in cocaine-exposed infants were directly associated with the ability of cocaine to produce abrupt changes in cerebral blood flow. In a study by Dixon and Bejar (1988), 41% of 32 infants exposed to cocaine during pregnancy suffered intracranial hemorrhage, cerebral infarction, and/or cerebral atrophy. These infants otherwise were judged healthy and had no obvious perinatal asphyxia/depression. Several smaller studies and single case reports seem to confirm that cocaine may extensively damage the developing fetal brain. Intrauterine and postnatal hypertension and vasoconstriction of the cerebral blood vessels appear to be the most likely causes of these dramatic and catastrophic findings.

In human newborns, the most commonly associated clinical symptoms of central nervous system pathology secondary to cocaine exposure are jitteriness, irritability, feeding difficulties, and increased muscle tone. These symptoms occur even in infants who do not have obvious radiologic changes in their brains. Chasnoff et al. (1985) and Eisen et al. (1991) have both noted significant depression of interactive behavior and a poor organizational response to environmental stimuli on the Brazelton Neonatal Behavior Assessment scale administered in the first 3 to 7 days of age. Comparison of animal data to human infant data is difficult because of the different maturational levels of the central nervous system at birth among different species studied. Studies in rats do seem to indicate increased habituation (simple learning) to environmental

stimuli and poor tolerance to stress when compared to rats who have not been exposed to intrauterine cocaine.

Long-term studies of infants exposed to cocaine during pregnancy have yet to be reported. Anecdotal reporting of older children with "worst case scenarios" of cocaine exposure dramatized in lay literature may make it difficult to discern the children who are more subtly affected, who may not have the entire constellation of cocaine-related abnormalities, and who may have slipped through the system without detection until reaching school age when learning deficits and/or attention deficit disorders may become more apparent.

The structural defects in organ systems other than the central nervous system that have been linked to cocaine abuse all probably fall into the category of vascular disruption syndromes. Traditionally, the fetus has been thought to be at risk for teratogenic effects of chemicals in the first 3 months following conception, when the majority of structural development is occurring. Intrauterine exposure to drugs, chemicals, or environmental teratogens is implied to cause interruption in the normal developmental sequences, leading to structural abnormalities. Recent evidence in animals and humans indicates that certain drugs, such as cocaine, may cause interruption of the intrauterine blood supply with a resultant disruption, or destruction, of previously formed and presumably normal organ systems. Hoyme et al. (1990) have suggested that the blood flow interruption is similarly related to the pharmacologic events that have been documented in adult humans, including brain hemorrhage accompanying rapid changes in systemic and cerebral blood flow, and hypoxia secondary to uterine, placental, or fetal vasoconstriction.

There are many factors that are believed to cause congenital structural defects in humans. Originally, any congenital deformity was thought to be secondary to an arrest of normal development of a structure at a certain embryologic stage. However, over the past several years, it has become evident that the causes of congenital structural defects can be divided into three categories:

> *Malformation:* A primary structural defect arising from a localized error in development (e.g., cleft lip/palate).
>
> *Deformation:* An alteration in shape or structure of a part that had already developed normally (e.g., clubfoot).
>
> *Disruption:* A structural defect resulting from destruction of a previously normally formed part (e.g., amputation of a digit or extremity).

Cocaine exposure during any stage of pregnancy has been identified as the cause of a disruptive pattern of congenital defects in human and animal studies. Intestinal obstruction secondary to vascular changes in the blood supply to the growing gut has been well documented. Limb reduction deficits (loss of digits, extremities, and so on) also have been documented in human and animal studies. Urinary tract defects have been variable. The most characteristic urinary tract anomaly associated with intrauterine cocaine exposure, the urethral obstruction syndrome (prune belly syndrome of lax abdominal musculature, outlet ureteral obstruction, and hydronephrosis) was postulated by Chasnoff, Chisum, and Kaplan (1988) to be directly related to fetal vascular spasm of the prostrate gland leading to changes in prostatic development with resultant urethral obstruction.

A study by Webster and Brown-Woodman (1990) seems to prove conclusively that the structural abnormalities associated with intrauterine cocaine exposure are due to the interruption of blood flow to developing, or previously developed, organ structures. Pregnant rats were injected with cocaine in mid and late gestation, after the bulk of organ development has already occurred. Forty-eight hours after exposure to the drug, the rat pups showed hemorrhages of the developing forelimbs and hindlimbs, the tail, the developing genitalia, upper lip, and cerebral hemispheres. The rat pups were then examined on the 21st day of gestation and were found to have limb reduction deficits, cleft lips, and cerebral changes that previously had been marked by the hemorrhages noted at 48 hours after cocaine exposure. The pattern of defects was very close to those seen in human infants.

The primary mechanism by which cocaine exerts its deleterious effects on the human infant is through its effect on fetal, placental, and uterine blood flow. Cocaine causes a spectrum of congenital anomalies dependent on the amount of diminished blood flow to the organ system involved, as well as the time of gestation at which the insult occurs. Cocaine clearly affects the fetus at variable stages of pregnancy, not just in the first trimester.

Recognition and Management of Cocaine-Abusing Mothers and Their Infants

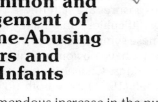

The tremendous increase in the numbers of pregnant women using cocaine has occurred so rapidly that medical and social service systems are being overwhelmed with the resultant problems. Research regarding the impact of cocaine on the developing fetus and the newborn is just emerging, but many questions remain unanswered. The issues of routes of administration, doses and timing, polydrug use, and the effects of cocaine on the mother and her infant, in addition to the unknown long-term ramifications on the neurobehavioral development in exposed babies need to be addressed; however, effective protocols for managing these problems must be developed before these issues can be resolved.

Unfortunately, there is not a single management strategy that will encompass all the variables inherent in the drug-using population of pregnant mothers and their newborns. Each health care provision system has to devise its own management protocol based on the factors that influence cocaine and other types of chemical abuse in that particular community. There are some general principles that can be tailored to effectively aid health care professionals in the recognition and management of these high-risk pregnancies and the resultant children. Often, the first indication of a problem is when a mother suddenly presents in labor with a history of minimal, or no, prenatal care. Table 2 shows some of the more common complications associated with pregnant cocaine-abusing women. If the mother presents to the health care facility under the obvious influence of drugs, the diagnosis easily may be confirmed by toxicology screening. More often than not, drug abuse is not clinically apparent, and the constellation of cocaine-associated problems must be elicited by history. If history taking can be done in a nonjudgmental and positive manner, many of these mothers will admit to the use of cocaine, or other illicit drugs, out of fear of the possible harmful effects on their infants. When suspicion of drug use is high, but the mother will not elicit the necessary information, other factors in the medical history may provide clues to drug abuse: late, or no, prenatal care; history of past chemical abuse; history of family violence; history of sexually transmitted diseases; history of removal of previous children from the home by social service agencies; and so on. Urine toxicology screens may be obtained only with the permission of the

Table 2. Maternal Complications Associated with Prenatal Cocaine Abuse

Lack of prenatal care
Poor general health
Poor nutritional habits
Inadequate weight gain
Increased incidence of sexually transmitted diseases
Hypertension and cardiac arrhythmias
Placental abruption
Premature delivery
Family violence
Psychological changes — depression

mother as a rule, and even if permission is granted, the outcome of the screen depends on when the last dose of cocaine, or other drugs, was administered. A negative drug screen does not rule out drug abuse in a mother where there is a high index of suspicion. Urine screens must be tailored to the drug-using population so that the most commonly abused drugs are routinely screened for. The metabolites of cocaine (ecgonine and benzoylecgonine) usually can be detected in the urine for 2 to 4 days following the last administered dose. Marijuana may be detected for up to 7 days after a single use in adults. Amphetamines may be present for 1 to 2 days following administration. Analysis of infant meconium stools has proved to be an effective screen of drug exposure, but while becoming more prevalent, it is not in general use. Analysis of maternal and infant hair samples has proven highly accurate and predictive of exposure over a much longer period than urine screening, but the analysis is expensive, time-consuming, and demands a level of expertise not available to the general public. It has not proven to be a cost-effective tool, but it is promising.

For the purpose of identifying infants at risk for intrauterine cocaine exposure, a positive urine screen in the mother or infant is adequate. However, many states require a positive infant urine screen for a definitive diagnosis before a report to protective, or social service, agencies is mandatory. If drug exposure is suspected, the infant should have urine screening as soon as possible after birth for the most reliable results. Rapid turnaround time of the screen from the laboratory is highly important, especially in these days of mandatory early discharges of mothers and their newborn infants from the hospital.

Knowledge of a mother's drug exposure, or positive urine toxicology screening, will identify the infant at risk for cocaine-related complications. Many infants are suspected clinically without strong evidence to support those suspicions. Careful assessment of the infant's physical state and behavioral characteristics in the nursery may provide further evidence of cocaine exposure during pregnancy, particularly if any of the constellation of problems named in Table 1 are seen. Intrauterine growth retardation may be diagnosed easily, but the causes of it are multiple; and a complete evaluation of the infant needs to be made before cocaine is implicated. Elevations of blood pressure, abnormalities of the cardiac rate and rhythm, and electrocardiographic changes consistent with diminished blood flow to the heart are not uncommonly seen in the cocaine-exposed infant and need to be differentiated from changes caused by other disorders. Intracranial hemorrhage may or may not be associated with clinical symptoms, but it should be evaluated for if there is suspicion of cocaine exposure because of the frequency with which it is reported to occur in these infants and the long-term ramifications it entails. Appropriate radiographic evaluation of the infant's central nervous system should be obtained prior to the infant's discharge. Limb reduction deficits are diagnosed easily on physical exam, but the causes must be differentiated from those associated with cocaine abuse and

those associated with other syndromes. Any congenital defects that could cause functional cosmetic problems should be evaluated thoroughly and treatment plans developed before discharge. Polydrug users are at high risk for sexually transmitted diseases (syphilis, gonorrhea, AIDS, chlamydia, and so on), and other significant diseases such as hepatitis B. Depending on the individual case, it may be warranted to evaluate the infant for any or all of these potentially dangerous infectious diseases — not only for the infant's sake, but for the protection of the health care workers involved.

It is important to evaluate the neurobehavioral state of infants at risk for cocaine exposure, even if they have none of the other findings in the clinical constellation. The cocaine-exposed infant tends to be very lethargic, poorly responsive, hypertonic, irritable when finally aroused, and jittery and disorganized in sleeping and feeding behavior. In awake states, these infants become hyperirritable if confronted with minimal environmental stimulation. They may cry inconsolably, or return to a sleep state, making maternal interactions very difficult and threatening to an already emotionally unstable mother. The lack of maternal interaction may lead to inappropriate and inadequate caretaking skills, particularly in a mother whose parenting skills may already be limited at best. Many of these infants are so difficult to feed that prolonged tube feeding is required before they "learn" how to eat — further isolating the mother from the infant.

Neurobehavioral changes may be quantitatively assessed in the Brazelton Neonatal Assessment and the Neonatal Abstinence Scale among others. Although seizures may not be clinically obvious, if they are suspected in the cocaine-exposed infant, an electroencephalogram should be obtained because of the reports of persistent EEG changes in these infants. Many of the neurobehavioral symptoms exhibited in the at-risk infant also are caused by a diversity of other conditions common in neonates — infections, metabolic derangements, asphyxia, and cardiorespiratory disease to name a few. It is important to rule out all other treatable causes of behavioral changes in the symptomatic newborn before assuming cocaine is the causative agent.

Prior to discharge, it is important to stress to the mother that these neurobehavioral abnormalities may persist for weeks or months. The mother, or significant other caregiver, must be trained to understand the infant's cues and how to respond to them appropriately. If the mother can be taught the early signs of overstimulation in her infant, she may be able to effectively avert excessive distress leading to the inconsolable crying and feeding problems that these infants often experience in the first months of life. Teaching a mother to recognize the distress signals and to provide the infant with a lesser degree of stimulation, or activity, to minimize the infant's response can be done by persons administering the behavioral assessment scales. Techniques such as swaddling, offering a pacifier, reducing environmental stimulation, and so on, should be taught to the mother prior to discharge and reinforced through home visits of health care professionals, or during the ongoing outpatient follow-up of the mother and infant. Techniques in feeding these infants need to be taught and reinforced to prevent maternal frustration. If a mother is suspected of continuing a lifestyle of cocaine, or polydrug abuse, breast feeding must be strongly discouraged because toxic levels of the drugs the mother ingests are excreted into the breast milk. If long-term follow-up is reasonably assured, and the mother agrees to remain drug free and submit to routine drug screening, then breast feeding is an alternative to bottle feeding that may help provide increased maternal-infant bonding.

The infant should be discharged only when all necessary assessments of cocaine-related problems have been completed. The noncompliant lifestyle of most cocaine abusers interferes with regular medical follow-up as an outpatient, so arrangements for providing home visitation by experienced health care professionals should be implemented. The infant should be nippling all feedings well and have an established weight gain. If there have been significant neurobehavioral changes in the nursery, the infant should show some signs of improvement prior to discharge; and the mother, or other caregiver, should be able to recognize the infant's distress signals and know what attempts to make to manage them. It must be determined that the infant will be discharged to a safe environment. If local laws and policies mandate reporting the infant of drug-abusing parents to the appropriate authorities, the procedure should be made clear to the parents. A strong recommendation to place the mother in an ongoing drug rehabilitation program should be made. The record of the infant's hospitalization should include the presumptive diagnosis of chemical abuse based on clinical suspicion, or positive drug screens. Observations of the infant's and parents' behavior should also be included in the chart in case legal intervention is necessary, or required by law to provide for the safety of the infant.

Once the decision to discharge the infant is reached and the social and legal ramifications are addressed, and the mother, or significant caregiver, has received appropriate training, care must be taken to ensure that a long-term follow-up program of the infant and mother by a physician and other health care professionals is in place and operative. During the first 2 months of life, the infant should be evaluated weekly, preferably by the same individual. Changes in neurobehavioral status in cocaine-exposed infants frequently occur between the second and fourth week of life. Sleeping and feeding patterns may be altered drastically, playing havoc with an already disturbed family. Appropriate intervention at this point may avert potential abuse and/or neglect. Some infants may require light sedation for management. Irritability sometimes can be managed by appropriate stress-relief techniques such as rocking, swaddling, and decreasing the amount of environmental stimulation.

The mother must understand that many of these infants develop an aversion to tactile stimulation and that excessive handling, jerky movements, frequent bathing, and so on, may all adversely affect the infant's behavior. During these periods, visiting health care professionals can assess the infant's condition, the mother's response to the infant's behavior, and the home situation in general. Important information then can be provided to the infant's physician and the legal system, if necessary.

In addition to the biochemical and anatomic damage done to the infant's developing central nervous system, many of the neurologic abnormalities associated with cocaine-exposed infants such as jitteriness, hypertonia, and excessive irritability interfere with the infant's ability to achieve its developmental milestones appropriately. For this reason, it is important that regular developmental follow-up be insisted upon; and if the infant demonstrates significant developmental delays, that an appropriate infant stimulation program be instituted. The child should receive developmental evaluations at least two to three times during the first year of life, two times during the second year, and yearly thereafter until at least age five. Subtle language, cognitive, and behavioral deficits may not become apparent until the child enters the primary grades in school, so a method of tracking these at-risk children should be developed to ensure early detection and treatment should a difficulty arise later in life.

In addition to infant intervention programs aimed at ensuring tracking of developmental milestones, children may require "family intervention programs" to create a more stable and supportive home atmosphere. Too often, the home environment of these cocaine-exposed children is chaotic and dysfunctional, making adjustments even more difficult for the at-risk child. Community child advocates are necessary to stimulate development and introduction of family oriented rehabilitation and intervention programs to meet the needs of these children. Communities and legislatures must be made aware of the tremendous potential risks involved in the future care of cocaine-exposed infants and their families. It is estimated that 500 million dollars is spent yearly just on taking care of cocaine-exposed infants in the immediate neonatal period. The costs can be multiplied astronomically when the long-term care of these children is contemplated. The funding of adequate prenatal care programs, drug rehabilitation programs for substance-abusing mothers, and the development of accurate drug-screening programs that are cost effective in populations of at-risk women is sure to be expensive initially, but will be more effective in meeting the needs of a future generation of cocaine-exposed children that otherwise could have been prevented. Educational programs on chemical abuse during pregnancy must be established at both the public and professional level. The public must be made to understand that any substance abuse by a woman during her pregnancy places her unborn child at significant medical risk and that this can occur even before pregnancy is diagnosed, or at any other stage of pregnancy. Professional education should focus on the ability to predict which women are at risk for substance abuse during pregnancy and to develop and administer programs to deal with them in a knowledgeable and supportive manner.

Conclusion

The number of infants born to cocaine-abusing mothers in the past few years has risen astronomically. Cocaine exposure during pregnancy has been linked directly to prematurity, intrauterine growth retardation, intracranial hemorrhage, and subsequent neurobehavioral deficits in addition to many other medical and social problems. Animal and human studies indicate that the drug can exert its effects at any stage of pregnancy by disrupting fetal vascular stability resulting in vasoconstriction and/or hemorrhage and leading to subsequent structural abnormalities. The difficulties involved in research studies regarding the effects of cocaine in pregnancy relate to the generally noncompliant population of cocaine abusers and the variability in dosage, timing, and route of cocaine exposure.

Although many of these cocaine-exposed infants are asymptomatic at birth, there is a recognizable constellation of associated problems that may lead health care professionals to the diagnosis. It is important that these infants be diagnosed and treated appropriately prior to discharge from the hospital to avert the possibility of future neglect and/or abuse, to alert the medical community and family that an infant may be at high risk for long-term developmental disability and neurobehavioral deficits, and to provide long-term follow-up of these infants.

The cost to society to provide funding for educational and rehabilitative programs for substance-abusing mothers is immense, but nothing compared to the cost of the long-term care of these children once they have been exposed to cocaine during pregnancy. Professional education programs are necessary to enlighten health care professionals about the risks of cocaine exposure to the developing fetus and newborn infant and how to recognize and treat this at-risk population. Chasnoff (1991, p. 120) stated:

"The most commonly missed diagnosis in obstetric and pediatric practice is maternal drug use in pregnancy, yet the long-term health and welfare of the children are at the greatest risk."

References

Chasnoff, I. J. (1989). Drug use and women: Establishing a standard of care. *Annals of New York Academy of Science, 562,* 208–210.

Chasnoff, I. J. (1991). Cocaine and pregnancy: Clinical and methodologic issues. *Clinics in Perinatology, 18,* 113–123.

Chasnoff, I. J., Burns, W. J., Schnoli, S. H., & Burns, K. A. (1985). Cocaine use in pregnancy. *New England Journal of Medicine, 313,* 666–669.

Chasnoff, I. J., Bussey, M. E., Savich, R., & Stack, M. S. (1986). Prenatal cerebral infarctions and maternal cocaine use. *Journal of Pediatrics, 108,* 456–459.

Chasnoff, I. J., Chisum, G. M., & Kaplan, W. E. (1988). Maternal cocaine use and genitourinary tract malformations. *Teratology, 37,* 201–204.

Chasnoff, I. J., Griffith, D. R. (1989). Cocaine: Clinical studies of pregnancy and the newborn. *Annals of the New York Academy of Science, 562,* 260–266.

Chasnoff, I. J., Landress, H. J., & Barrett, M. E. (1990). The prevalence of illicit drug or alcohol use during pregnancy and discrepancies in mandatory reporting in Pinellas County, Florida. *New England Journal of Medicine, 322,* 1202–1206.

Chouteau, M., Numerow, P. B., & Leppert, P. (1988). The effect of cocaine abuse on birth weight and gestational age. *Obstetrics & Gynecology, 72,* 351–354.

Dison, S. D., & Bejar, R. (1988). Brain lesions in cocaine and methamphetamine exposed neonates. *Pediatric Research, 23,* 405A.

Doberczak, T. M., Shanzer, S., Senie, R. T., & Kandall, S. R. (1988). Neonatal neurologic and electroencephalographic effects of intrauterine cocaine exposure. *Journal of Pediatrics, 113,* 354–358.

Eisen, L. N., Field, T. M., Bandstra, E. S., Roberts, J. P., Morrow, C., Larson, S. K., & Steele, B. M. (1991). Perinatal cocaine effects on neonatal stress behavior and performance on the Brazelton Scale. *Pediatrics, 88,* 477–480.

Hoyme, H. E., Jones, K. L., Dixon, S. D., Jewet, T., Hanson, J. W., Robinson, L. K., Msall, M. E., & Allanson, J. E. (1990). Perinatal cocaine exposure and fetal vascular disruption. *Pediatrics, 85,* 743–747.

Hume, R. F., O'Donnell, K. J., Stanger, C. L., Killam, A. P., & Gingras, J. L. (1989). In utero cocaine exposure: Observations of fetal behavioral state may predict neonatal outcome. *American Journal of Obstetrics & Gynecology, 161,* 685–690.

Kramer, L. D., Locke, G. E., Ogunyemi, A., & Nelson, L. (1990). Neonatal cocaine related seizures. *Journal of Child Neurology, 5,* 60–64.

Little, B. B., Snell, L. M., & Klein, V. R. (1989). Cocaine abuse during pregnancy: Adverse perinatal outcome. *American Journal of Obstetrics & Gynecology, 73,* 157–160.

Madden, J. D., Payne, T. F., & Miller, S. (1986). Maternal cocaine use and effect on the newborn. *Pediatrics, 77,* 209–211.

Webster, W. S., & Brown-Woodman, P. D. (1990). Cocaine as a cause of congenital malformation of vascular origin: Experimental evidence in the rat. *Teratology, 41,* 689–697.

Woods, J. R., Plessinger, M. A., Scott, K., & Miller, R. K. (1989). Prenatal cocaine exposure: A sheep model for cardiovascular evaluation.

Address correspondence to:
Charles C. MacDonald, M.D., Special Care Nursery, St. Mary's Medical Center, 3700 Washington Avenue, Evansville, IN 47750

Working with Families of Drug-Exposed Children: Three Model Programs

Linda S. Crites, Ph.D., LCSW
Baltimore City Head Start HIV Project

Kayleen L. Fischer, M.S., CCC SLP
Intervention with Parents and Children Together, Inc.

Mary McNeish-Stengel, M.S.W., LCSW
Our Friends' Place

Clare J. Siegel, M.S.
Coordinator, Baltimore City Head Start HIV Project
Baltimore, Maryland

Families of drug-exposed children present multiple service needs beyond the scope of early intervention programs. However, close coordination among agencies providing a broad spectrum of services is necessary to maintain family integrity and to address the developmental needs of the children

In Baltimore, Maryland, there are three programs that work with these families. One of the programs has primarily an educational focus, one of the programs focuses primarily on supportive and therapeutic services to parents, and the third project focuses primarily on therapeutic services to children.

Background

With rates of substance abuse climbing, especially among undereducated, poor, inner city, disadvantaged populations, children born to these environments face a wide range of threats to their physical, cog-nitive, emotional, and social development. Considerable controversy exists around the developmental and behavioral effects on the infant who is prenatally exposed to drugs. The types of drugs used, amount and method of use, and timing of use are drug-related factors that contribute to the pres-

Infant-Toddler Intervention.
The Transdisciplinary Journal (Vol. 2, No. 1, pp. 13–23)
© 1992, Singular Publishing Group, Inc.

ence or absence of adverse effects on the child exposed in utero (Cole, Jones, & Sadofsky, 1990). Additionally, adequate research efforts to reliably determine the developmental impact of specific drugs is undermined by polysubstance abuse, poor maternal health, and lack of prenatal care. Preexisting and ongoing effects of intergenerational family dysfunction, chemical abuse, poverty, and environmental deprivation also complicate efforts to delineate the consequences of substance use and abuse alone (Cole et al., 1990).

Although the nature of the use of illegal substances precludes certainty of accurate and complete statistics, all indications are that "the incidence and prevalence of perinatal drug exposure is substantial and rising" (Cole et al., 1990, p. 5). A recent nationwide survey estimated that 11% of all newborns in the United States are exposed to illegal drugs during the prenatal and perinatal period (Gittler & McPherson, 1990). Statistics focusing on adolescents are even more frightening. A 1989 study at Boston City Hospital found that slightly over half of the pregnant adolescents participating used alcohol during their pregnancies; one third had used marijuana; and almost one fifth had used cocaine while pregnant (Amaro, Zuckerman, & Cabral, 1989).

Because the explosion of drug use during pregnancy has been so recent, well-designed, longitudinal studies of the long-term effects on children are virtually nonexistent. Shorter term investigations have found that neonates who have suffered drug exposure are more likely to be premature, small for gestational age, and more vulnerable to neonatal morbidity, mortality, and to display disruptions in normal neonatal motor, interactional, and state control abilities (Schneider, Griffith, & Chasnoff, 1989). However, some research has indicated that these problems subside within several months, whereas other studies have found that deleteri-

ous effects of drug exposure continue. Generally, investigations using standardized measures of infant development have revealed little difference between babies who were drug exposed and those who were not. No typical profile of drug-affected children has been defined, yet subtle temperamental and behavioral difficulties have been identified in these children (Cole et al., 1990).

Despite the inconsistencies in research findings, broad trends in less formal, clinical data suggest that there is a range of vulnerabilities that may result from intrauterine drug exposure. Infants drug exposed during gestation most frequently are reported to be irritable and hypersensitive to external stimuli; to exhibit feeding and sleeping difficulties; to have tone, reflex, and movement abnormalities; and to produce decreased vocalization (Weston, Ivins, Zuckerman, Jones, & Lopez, 1989). Drug-exposed toddlers and preschoolers often are distracted more easily, overstimulated, emotionally labile, and they may exhibit disruptions in motor and language development and attachment behavior and social interaction (Weston et al., 1989).

These later problems also may result from or be exacerbated by the psychological stressors and environmental problems that have an impact on the child and family. Patterns of intergenerational substance abuse and family dysfunction in the background of the substance-abusing mother further compound the risk for parenting problems. Ongoing substance abuse will certainly increase the risk for child neglect or abuse resulting in developmental and emotional damage. Moreover, growing rates of HIV infection in substance-abusing and heterosexual groups and the resultant increase in perinatal transmission present additional medical, developmental, and social dangers for these children. Loss of a parent to ongoing substance abuse or illness and death from AIDS may ultimately result in abandonment and out-of-home placement of the child. A succession of foster placements brought on by parental crises, or by the child's developmental or emotional difficulties, further increases the risk of exacerbating the child's problems and hinders attempts at remediation.

Service Needs of Families and Children

Several factors contribute to the necessity for considering the family unit as a whole when providing services to children in general, and specifically to those who have been prenatally drug exposed. Longstanding debates in the field of child development and child welfare have questioned the effects of separating the child from the family, and based on years of study, the prevailing attitude among child specialists today is that the child should be maintained within the family if at all possible. Respect for parental rights and concerns about emotional damage to the child due to separation from the family have promoted a societal commitment to preserving families and preventing family disintegration. On a more practical side, appropriate foster families are increasingly difficult to recruit, especially for children with special needs. Group care for young children has long been recognized as inadequate to meet the needs for care and nurturing of the very young child. Moreover, the monetary costs of appropriate alternative care have been found to exceed the financial costs of providing support and remediation resources to the family unit. If maintaining a child in the family is to be a goal, any program that is going to meet the child's needs must address family problems as well.

As previously suggested, the needs of children who have been prenatally drug abused vary with the child, based on his or her unique history. The type and extent of drug exposure, as well as complicating perinatal events and neonatal illnesses, such as prematurity or intracranial hemorrhage may all affect the developmental status and potential of the child. Additionally, infants compromised by substance abuse in utero, poor prenatal care, drug withdrawal, or other neonatal complications are less likely to respond appropriately to and interact with even the most nurturing and skillful caregiver.

Clinical as well as research evidence demonstrates that, for mothers actively using drugs or going through withdrawal during the prenatal or perinatal periods, relating to and caring for their newborn is frequently overshadowed by other concerns. However, it also has been demonstrated that substance abuse treatment for the mother positively influences the social and developmental capacity of the children. For this reason, the provision of substance abuse treatment is crucial to any plan aimed at establishing an environment that promotes the development of the child. Unfortunately, there is a seriously limited availability of publicly funded drug treatment programs, most have long waiting lists, and few actually admit pregnant women. Further, women with children have the additional problem of securing child care while in residential treatment programs (Gittler & McPherson, 1990).

Psychotherapy and other supportive social services also are integral to service plans for families with drug-exposed children. Many parents with substance abuse problems come from dysfunctional backgrounds in which they were emotionally deprived and which have left serious emotional scars. These parents often have learned inappropriate patterns of interacting with others in general, and of parenting specifically. As a result, psychotherapy for the adult with substance abuse problems is an important element of treatment, and it often involves a substantial amount of reparenting. Especially for individuals affected by intergenerational substance abuse, creating a positive role model for parenting is every bit as important as dealing with the psychological sequelae of being raised in a dysfunctional family.

The infant's impaired interactive ability coupled with the likelihood of the mother's diminished caregiving capacity increases the potential for major problems in maternal-child interaction, particularly as that interaction is related to formation of attachment, development of the child, and potential for child abuse and neglect. Because of the reciprocal nature of the interaction and relationship between parent and child, a multidisciplinary, early intervention model is most appropriate for working with families where substance abuse has an impact on the child's development. Early intervention programs integrate development-promoting experiences with needed therapeutic interventions from physical and occupational therapists and speech and language specialists. Parent training focused on understanding the child's needs, setting realistic expectations of the child, and appropriate parent-child interaction is a significant component of many early intervention programs.

As mentioned, in addition to problems directly related to the child's development and the relationship between parent and child, families affected by substance abuse face a multitude of psychosocial stressors that may detract from their abilities to provide an appropriate and nurturing environment. Employment and financial problems are often a cause as well as an effect of substance abuse, and often the most basic needs of the family, such as food and shelter, are inadequately met. The absence of appropriate child care alternatives may further hinder the efforts of mothers raising their children alone and other parents who may need additional education or job training. Legal concerns resulting from a family member's drug-related activities can cause further financial and emotional drains on the family.

Substance-abusing individuals and their families are subjected to considerable social stigma and rejection, especially when the chemically dependent person is a mother or a pregnant woman. Without a clear understanding of and sensitivity to the complex web of stresses and problems associated with substance use and abuse, service providers may be unable to overcome their own frustrations and prejudices about working with these families. Families affected by chemical addiction often bear the brunt of negative attitudes and lack of respect from service providers as well as a lack of warmth, caring, and understanding (Pollack, Spiegel, Mayers, & Marshall, 1988). Programs serving drug-exposed children must work in concert with the family and respect parents' views of the child's needs and family's problems. Without collaboration with the family, underlying psychosocial problems will go unaddressed and will continue to interfere with the family's ability to provide appropriate care of the child. Programs must be extremely careful to assure coordination of services, given the multiple and varied range of service needs, which may include developmental therapies for the child, supportive psychotherapy for parents, parent training, substance abuse treatment, job training, housing and financial assistance for the family, in addition to the usual health and educational needs of families. Clearly, no one program can provide for all of these families' needs, and, therefore, a variety of programs will be involved. Consequently, frequent and open communication among agencies working with the family is vital to avoid service gaps as well as overlaps. It is also important to designate a primary coordinating agency and person with whom the family connects. Ultimately, the primary service coordinator, or case manager, may serve as an advisor to the family and as an advocate with the service system, so that the family is not too overwhelmed to utilize services effectively.

Program Descriptions

In Baltimore, three model programs work collaboratively to address the multiple service needs of families affected by substance abuse. Intervention with Parents and Children Together, Inc. focuses primarily on providing therapeutic services to children who are developmentally delayed, while Our Friends' Place focuses on supportive and therapeutic services to parents. The Pediatric HIV Project of the Baltimore City Head Start program is targeted toward families affected by HIV infection. However, close coordination among these programs, and with other agencies in the community, provides families with an organized constellation of services to meet their needs.

PACT

Intervention with Parents and Children Together, Inc. (PACT) began as a Title V demonstration project in Baltimore in 1978. Originally, the program was operated through the University of Maryland School of Medicine's Department of Pediatrics. However, after having demonstrated its effectiveness, the program became a private, nonprofit agency in 1981. As one of Maryland's first early intervention programs, PACT's goals were focused on serving infants and toddlers who were at high risk for developmental delays. Today, PACT's mission is to promote the development of young children with special needs ranging from developmental delays to cerebral palsy, from mental retardation to HIV infection. While some of these children's special needs are the result of prenatal alcohol or drug abuse by their parents, by virtue of their special

needs or psychosocial stressors in the family, all are considered to be at risk for abuse or neglect. Each of PACT's programs promotes the participation of the family and operates within the context of the community. Most often, referrals for program services come from local medical facilities, private pediatricians, social service agencies, or directly from parents themselves.

Like many early intervention programs, PACT uses a multidisciplinary team approach to the provision of therapy services and family support; this team consists of physical, occupational, and speech therapists and social workers. A plan for therapeutic intervention is developed by the team, and a case manager is chosen from among the various team members. The role of the case manager is to monitor the provision of services within the program, to connect the family to outside resources as needed, to provide family support, and to facilitate planning for transition to subsequent programming when developmentally or age appropriate.

Several different types of therapeutic programs are available to children and families from PACT. In the center-based program, child and parent/caregiver receive individualized therapeutic intervention on a weekly basis. Child and parent participate together in therapy so that the parent/caregiver can learn about the child's developmental needs and how to relate appropriately to the child. Care is taken to address special needs of the child along with parent problems that might hinder interaction between parent and child in the home environment. Therapists and parent work together to establish developmentally realistic goals for the child and family. Written as well as verbal instruction in therapeutic techniques is given to parents so they can be carried over to the home setting.

Parents In Action (PIA), a special parenting program for parents with cognitive limitations, was begun in 1987 to enhance the limited parent's ability to provide appropriate care for the child. PACT's goal of decreasing the heightened risk of child abuse and neglect found in children with special needs has also been a primary concern of this program. The program teaches parents limit setting with their children, ways to provide enriched learning environment and creative play experiences for the child, and methods for building self-esteem. Because of the increased risk of substance abuse in individuals who are cognitively limited, this program incorporates education focused on substance abuse prevention as well as coordination with substance abuse treatment programs and other resources for parents enrolled in PIA. Although not the primary focus of this program, speech, occupational, and physical therapy are available to the child if needed and appropriate.

In 1988, PACT received a substantial grant from the UPS Foundation to initiate a day care program for infants and toddlers with developmental handicaps requiring ongoing therapeutic services. A major goal of this program is to integrate and mainstream children who are developmentally impaired with children who do not have special needs. Occupational, speech, and physical therapy are available to the child within the day care setting; consequently, parents are able to maintain work or training schedules without the constant need to take time off to take children to therapy appointments. Parents involved in this program are required to participate at least once a week, so that they can take part in therapeutic and education programs and to allow for follow-up of the family's progress.

For families who are experiencing more serious social problems or mental health difficulties, the Therapeutic Nursery Program was established in 1990. The Therapeutic Nursery provides both therapeutic intervention for special needs children along with intensive work with parents around educational, employment, and career issues. Structured on a play group model, which meets two mornings per week, this program creates a setting where therapeutic play with children and parents conjointly encourages parenting skills and child development, while helping parent and child learn to enjoy interacting together. In addition to parenting skills training, mental health services are integral to this program. One-to-one counseling with the parent addresses self-esteem and relationship issues, as well as other life stresses including substance abuse. Close coordination with substance abuse treatment programs further strengthens the parent's effort to prevent or combat drug or alcohol addiction and to prevent relapse.

In addition to the main site, the Therapeutic Nursery has a satellite operating within a local shelter for homeless families. This satellite provides early educational and play experiences for the children throughout the day, and frees parents to look for work and/or housing, comfortable in knowing that their children are safe and receiving good care.

Each of the programs within PACT can provide special assistance to families with substance abuse problems. When working with parents recovering from alcohol or drug addiction, the staff is especially concerned with keeping therapeutic expectations realistic. Guidelines and instructions for interacting with their children are concrete and explicit. Small, incremental goals are established so that parents will not become overwhelmed and more vulnerable to relapse. Educational information on drug and alcohol use and abuse and the prenatal effects on children, as well as on the user, are available to all parents on a one-to-one basis or in a classroom setting. Additionally, the case management model assures close coordination with outside substance abuse treatment programs working with the families.

Our Friends' Place

Our Friends' Place (OFP) is a community-based family support program sponsored by St. Jerome's Head Start Center in Baltimore. Established in 1985, OFP was founded on the philosophy that the family stresses that contribute to the risk of child abuse and neglect could be reduced by the provision of resources such as parenting education, a consistent social support system, and respite from the demands of child care. Initially, an informal "coffee and donut" program was set up, where mothers could have coffee together and discuss parenting problems with a trained counselor while their children received care from the center's staff. A range of ongoing psychosocial problems with which these parents were wrestling soon emerged; these problems included domestic violence and substance abuse and often were related to their own sexual or physical abuse as children. Subsequently, the scope of services provided by the program was expanded to address intergenerational abuse and neglect, substance abuse, and poverty.

Today, the mission of OFP is to prevent and ameliorate the effects of child maltreatment, and the program serves the southern and southwestern sections of Baltimore, areas that have been found to have the highest rates of child abuse and neglect in this city. OFP provides nurturing, educational programs, and supportive services for both children and parents at risk. Clients are referred from a variety of systems — medical, social service, and judicial. In particular, judges and family court officials may refer parents convicted of child abuse as an alternative to incarceration.

Currently, all of the parents served by the program are women; most are single heads of household. All of these women have at some time in their lives been the victims of some form of abuse or neglect and, consequently, present with many of the resulting difficulties abused individuals face. Most clients enter the program with low self-esteem and depression. They often have deep-seated and unresolved anger related to their own experiences of loss, separation, and abandonment. Not surprisingly, most of these women have abused their children or allowed them to be abused.

The vast majority of these clients have attempted to escape their predicaments through alcohol and/or drugs. Most of the children have some type of developmental or emotional problem resulting either directly from the mother's substance use or indirectly from psychosocial problems associated with substance-abusing lifestyles.

Multimodal therapy and educational training are provided for parents, 20 hours per week, in a home-like setting in which parent-child bonding is facilitated. At OFP, mothers are required to be on-site with their children 5 hours a day, 4 days per week. Each week at OFP, mothers receive individual psychotherapy and supervised parent-child interaction time within the context of a 5-hour weekly parenting seminar. Through role modeling as well as through supervising structured dyadic interactions between parent and child, teachers, child care providers, and counseling staff provide instruction to parents on how to nurture and relate to their children. Psychotherapeutic and psychoeducational groups are ongoing, including groups on substance abuse, sexual assault, domestic violence, health issues, and economic self-sufficiency. Clients also have an opportunity to attend literacy and GED classes, as well as to participate in structured recreational activities.

While mothers are involved in their daily activities, their children attend one of three on-site Head Start classrooms. Consistent with the Head Start framework, infants, toddlers, and preschoolers receive education, stimulation, and socialization. When developmental or behavioral concerns surface, children are evaluated by a physical, occupational, or speech therapist, education specialist, or physician as appropriate. If delays are identified, therapeutic services are provided on-site.

Women who have temporarily lost custody of their children also may be referred to OFP's "Foster Care Reunification" program. In this program, infants, toddlers, and preschoolers placed in foster care can attend the center two to four times per week. During this time, mothers visit with their children under supervised conditions; mothers receive instruction and counseling aimed at developing necessary skills for caring for the child appropriately, so that he or she can be returned home to the parent's care.

OFP also operates a "crisis nursery" that allows parents in the community, as well as in the regular OFP program, to obtain respite from their children or emergency child care while tending to problems such as eviction notices, utility cut-offs, or pursuing ex parte orders within the courts.

Program evaluation indicates that the effectiveness of the OFP program is related to the intensity and duration of the working relationship with parents, as well as to the multimodal range of interventions that are customized to serve individual parents. Within the OFP framework, mothers are able to build a strong support network of women and staff who are drug-free, and can regularly engage in interaction with others that fosters self-esteem and personal empowerment.

The Baltimore City Head Start Pediatric HIV Project

The Baltimore City Head Start Pediatric HIV Project began in 1988 as a grant-funded project intended to provide educational and supportive services to children in families affected by HIV and to promote a network of services to these children and families. National and local statistics show that approximately 75% of children infected with HIV are born to mothers who were infected through their own intravenous drug use or through sexual activity with a drug-abusing partner. Statistics from the Pediatric HIV Project show a similar majority from families where substance abuse is a significant issue (Crites & Siegel, 1990).

As an extension of the existing Head Start program in Baltimore, the HIV project is based on a family centered, community-based, interagency service delivery model. The main focus of the project is to provide early intervention and preschool educational services to children with HIV infection, who are at risk for HIV infection, or those whose mother has tested positive for HIV. Founded on a philosophy of mainstreaming, the program seeks to integrate children into the regular Head Start classrooms whenever possible, and experience has confirmed the belief that the programming needs of children affected by HIV are not substantially different from the needs of other children being served by Head Start and other preschool programs.

For children under age three and for those whose medical condition is more serious, services to the child are provided at the specialized Head Start Support Center or through a home-based model. For children 3 years and older, the project team facilitates the educational placement into one of the approximately 14 Head Start programs in Baltimore City. As with all Head Start programs, promoting development and positive learning experiences is a major objective of the HIV Project. Maintaining health and preventing or delaying loss of skills is of foremost concern, and close attention is given to all aspects of the child's development, including fine and gross motor skills, cognition, language, and social skills. Educational activities are provided according to a developmental model and are adapted to meet the child's individual needs. Referrals for speech and language, physical, and occupational therapy evaluations are made on an individual basis when concerns about the child's development arise, and ongoing therapy is provided within the Head Start program when needed.

In addition to receiving preschool programming for the child, all parents are eligible to participate in educational and recreational activities through the regular Head Start programs citywide. Families may continue to receive specialized supportive services through the HIV project if they desire. These support services are provided by a team that may include early childhood teachers and assistants and parent liaisons, and staff is available to the family on a 24-hour on-call basis. Parent liaisons assist parents with obtaining medical and social services, as well as providing guidance and assistance with interpersonal problems. Helping families during crisis periods as well as in obtaining concrete services such as housing, financial assistance, and food are an ongoing role for the project parent liaisons. In addition, formal and informal counseling addresses issues of denial and fears of disclosure. Individual counseling is available to parents, and education and support groups offer help to parents with problems ranging from nutrition to discipline. The project coordinator, who is an early intervention specialist, and a social work consultant provide ongoing supervision and consultation for the team, as well as working with family members directly when warranted. Issues related to substance abuse and HIV infection are addressed, and a number of mothers involved in the project are enrolled in substance abuse treatment programs. Additional consultation is provided to the team by Baltimore City Head Start specialists for Handicapped Services, Health, Social Services, and Parent Involvement.

Communication and cooperation with other agencies involved with the family are essential to the coordinated supervision of services to the child, and project staff work closely with medical and health providers, foster care agencies, and the local departments of social services and education, in addition to other early intervention programs.

HIV education and awareness training on transmission, the medical and psychosocial effects of HIV on the child and family, and societal attitudes and stigma are an ongoing component of the program. Because of the minimal risk of transmission in day care and school settings, no modifications in routine infection control procedures traditionally required in all Head Start programs were necessary. However, from early in the project, Head Start staff received training and education aimed at reducing fears and prejudices resulting from misinformation and misconceptions about children and adults affected by HIV. Additionally, parent education sessions on HIV issues have helped to minimize community discomfort about integrating children with HIV infection into centers and to educate the community about HIV prevention. Head Start is currently in the process of instituting substance abuse education program-wide, and the HIV project will be working collaboratively with centers to augment this training.

Now in its third year, the Pediatric HIV project has received permanent Head Start funding. In addition to expanding services to an increasing number of families affected by HIV, a community interagency network, the Baltimore Pediatric AIDS Care Consortium (PACC), has developed as a result of the project. Virtually every agency providing services to children affected by HIV and their families within the Baltimore area is represented on the PACC. Regular meetings create a forum in which agencies can communicate and share information about the latest developments in medical treatments and social services. Unmet service needs and service gaps in the community are identified and, with the assistance of the legislative subcommittee, member agencies keep abreast of current legislation affecting families affected by HIV and providers who serve them.

Guidelines for Program Development

Based on the combined experiences of these innovative programs, several guidelines for program development can be established.

First and foremost, the program should address an existing need for services within the community. Whether formal or informal, a needs assessment should be conducted within the community. Consultation with existing resources and service providers, as well as directly with families, will help to confirm or refute assumptions or misconceptions about service needs. For example, current needs assessment in Baltimore indicate that while specialized therapeutic programs are available for children with special needs, regular full-time day care for these children is still lacking.

Programs also must have a circumscribed scope; given the multiple problems facing families affected by substance abuse, it is unrealistic for any program to attempt to meet all of the service needs these families present. Consequently, an integrated approach to coordination with existing agencies and programs is likely to be most viable. Additionally, community involvement and support is especially vital to program development in current times of funding cutbacks. Funding sources are unwilling to subsidize programs that duplicate existing services unnecessarily, or those that do not have a demonstrable probability of cost-

effective success. Program developers need to be skillful at educating communities about local programming needs and at dovetailing goals with priorities of funding sources.

As previously discussed, programs need to take a family focus to promote stabilization of the home environment. Family involvement is as important to the process of program development as it is to the actual provision of services. Without the families' perspective on what services are needed and will be used, services will not be designed in a way to optimize utilization. Program operating hours, location, and potential stigma associated with use are all factors that require family input.

Finally, appropriate training of program staff is critical to success. Too often it is assumed that professionals are equipped to deal with special populations such as families affected by substance abuse. Although the developmental needs of these children and the service needs of the families may not differ substantially in content from other special populations, it is clear that the scope of services needed may be vast. Moreover, staff education and training may be even more important to address prejudices, misconceptions, frustrations, and negative attitudes about families with substance abuse problems.

References

Amaro, H., Zuckerman, B., & Cabral, H. (1989). Drug use among adolescent mothers: Profile of risk. *Pediatrics, 84,* 144–150.

Cole, C. K., Jones, M., & Sadofsky, G. (1990). Working with children at risk due to prenatal substance abuse. *PRISE Reporter, 21,* 5.

Crites, L. S., & Siegel, C. (1990, May/June). Improving quality of life for youngsters with HIV. *Children Today, 19* (3), 24–27.

Gittler, J., & McPherson, M. (1990, July/August). Prenatal substance abuse. *Children Today, 14* (4), 3–7.

Pollack, H., Spiegel, L., Mayers, A., & Marshall, F. (1988). Psychosocial aspects of HIV infection in children: The complexity of care. In *Feelings and Their Medical Significance* (pp. 9–14). Columbus, OH: Ross Laboratories.

Schneider, J. W., Griffith, D. R., & Chasnoff, I. J. (1989). Infants exposed to cocaine in utero: Implications for developmental assessment and intervention. *Infants and Young Children, 2,* 25–36.

Weston, D. R., Ivins, B., Zuckerman, B., Jones, C., & Lopez, R. (1989). Drug exposed babies: Research and clinical issues. *Zero to Three, 9* (5), 1–7.

Address correspondence to:
Kayleen L. Fischer, M. S., Intervention with PACT, Inc., 106 E. Chase Street, Baltimore, MD 21202

Audiologic Findings in Infants Born to Cocaine-Abusing Mothers

Barbara Cone-Wesson, Ph.D.

Department of Otolaryngology – Head and Neck Surgery
University of Southern California
School of Medicine
Los Angeles, California

Paul Wu, M.D.

Department of Pediatrics – Division of Neonatology
University of Southern California
School of Medicine
Los Angeles, California

The purpose of this article is to review literature relating to maternal cocaine use as a risk factor for infant auditory system impairment or abnormal development. Cocaine has been shown to be acutely neuro- and ototoxic in experimental animals. Maternal cocaine use affects neonatal neurologic status as well as neurodevelopment. Auditory evoked potential tests, specifically, auditory brainstem responses (ABRs), have been used to determine auditory system effects of maternal cocaine use. The ABR studies showed that there is no increased risk of hearing impairment among full-term normal birthweight infants born to cocaine-abusing mothers. The ABR studies further show that central auditory nervous system function is abnormal in cocaine-exposed neonates. These results argue for the existence of subtle differences in brainstem auditory system function, even when peripheral auditory system function is normal. Neurodevelopmental insult caused by maternal cocaine use suggests that these infants should be targeted for speech, language, and cognitive assessment at the earliest possible time.

Introduction

One goal of pediatric audiology is to detect auditory system impairment in early infancy. Auditory system impairment includes any disease or lesion, congenital or acquired, that could cause hearing impairment or central auditory nervous system (CANS) dysfunction. There are risk criteria known to be associated with infant hearing impairment (Joint

Infant-Toddler Intervention.
The Transdisciplinary Journal (Vol. 2, No. 1, pp. 25–35)
© 1992, Singular Publishing Group, Inc.

Committee on Infant Hearing, 1991), and some of these risk factors also are associated with delayed or abnormal neurologic (and possibly CANS) development. The precarious developmental status of infants born to women using illicit drugs led us to ask whether these infants are at risk for impaired auditory system function. The purpose of this article is to review the literature relating to maternal cocaine use as a risk factor for infant auditory system impairment or abnormal development. Several studies to determine the presence and extent of auditory system impairment in infants born to cocaine-abusing mothers (ICAMs) will be described. Directions for future research will be included.

Auditory Evoked Potentials (AEPs) for Infant Assessment

Infant auditory system function can be sampled using behavioral and electrophysiological techniques (Kile & Beauchaine, 1991). At this time, there are no published studies that have tested ICAMs' auditory function using behavioral methods. The effects of cocaine upon newborn auditory system function have, however, been measured using auditory evoked potentials (Cone-Wesson & Spingarn, 1990; Salamy, Eldredge, Anderson, & Bull, 1990; Shih, Cone-Wesson, & Reddix, 1988). It is necessary, then, to briefly describe how auditory evoked potentials (AEPs) are used to measure infant auditory system function.

AEP measurements are sensitive and specific indicators of auditory system abnormality. AEPs are changes in brain activity elicited by sound. They are recorded using modified electroencephalographic techniques and computer averaging. AEPs can

be measured from every level of the auditory nervous system from cochlea to auditory cortex. The auditory brainstem response (ABR), one of the AEPs, has become an integral part of the audiologic and neurologic test battery for young infants (Picton, Taylor, Durieux-Smith, & Edwards, 1986). The ABR reflects the neural response of the eighth nerve and brainstem auditory pathway (Møller, Janneta, & Møller, 1981). Determination of the lowest signal level needed to elicit an ABR and changes in the ABR latency (timing) can be used to detect hearing impairment, and estimate its severity (Galambos & Hecox, 1978). Other measures of the ABR, including the relative latency of individual response components (inter-peak latency), can be used to detect brainstem impairment (Stockard & Rossiter, 1977). The ABR has also been used as a measure of auditory nervous system development in both normal infants (Hecox & Burkhard, 1982) and those at risk for developmental delay (Salamy, 1984). The ABR is reliably recorded in neonates, even in premature newborns (Rottveel, Colon, Stegman, & Visco, 1987a, 1987b).

Definition of Auditory System Impairment

The basic types of peripheral hearing impairment were described recently in this journal by Kile and Beauchaine (1991). Hearing impairment caused by disease or lesion of the external, middle, inner ear or auditory nerve is understood as a loss of sensitivity for sound. The frequency range of impairment, as well as the degree of impairment can be quantified. Hearing impairment can be described and quantified using AEP techniques, and the ABR is especially useful in this area, as described above.

Auditory evoked potentials are used to detect lesions or dysfunction in the central auditory nervous system (Starr, 1977; Stockard & Rossiter, 1977). Evoked potential findings such as prolonged latencies, diminished amplitudes, or absence of evoked response components can be related directly to abnormalities in structure or function of the CANS. It stands to reason that the integrity of the CANS is a requisite for auditory perceptual skills and oral-language learning. A correlation between abnormalities in the CANS (shown by ABRs) and complex perceptual skills has not been firmly established yet. In this article, we will refer to ABR measures that indicate abnormal or delayed maturation of brainstem (central) auditory processing. We will call these "central auditory system impairments." The reader needs to understand that these functional abnormalities may not result from obvious perceptual abnormalities.

Cocaine Effects on the Newborn

Estimates of drug use among pregnant women are alarming: studies show that up to 10% of infants born in metropolitan county hospitals have been exposed to cocaine in utero (Little, Snell, Palmore, & Gilstrap, 1988). The morbidity and mortality of substance abuse has been well documented. For cocaine-using pregnant women, the risk of morbidity and mortality extends to their infants (Bingol, Fuchs, Diaz, Store, & Gromish, 1987; Chasnoff, Burns, Schnoll, & Burns, 1985; Oro & Dixon, 1987).

Fetal alcohol syndrome (FAS) is an example of substance abuse during pregnancy resulting in craniofacial anomalies, mental and growth retardation, and developmental delays (Clarren & Smith, 1978). A clinical syndrome has not been described yet for the effects of maternal cocaine abuse. However, it is clear that the developing fetus is compromised. Maternal cocaine use has been related to low birthweight, prematurity, and intrauterine growth retardation (Bingol et al, 1987; Chasnoff et al, 1985; Choutea, Namerow, & Leppert, 1988; Oro & Dixon, 1987; Ryan, Ehrlich, & Finnegan, 1987). Indicators of neonatal integrity, such as Apgar scores and head circumference are depressed (Oro & Dixon, 1987; Ryan, Ehrlich, & Finnegan, 1987). The birth defect rate is increased among ICAMs. Heart, skull (Bingol et al, 1987), genitourinary tract malformations (Chasnoff, Chisum, & Kaplan, 1988), and other defects thought to be caused by fetal vascular disruptions (Hoyme et al., 1990) have been documented.

It is notable that low birthweight, prematurity, and low Apgar scores are associated with increased rates of hearing impairment in infancy (Carter & Wilkening, 1991). Infant low birthweight and prematurity cause many medical complications including respiratory distress and increased susceptability to infection, that lead to treatment with ototoxic drugs. These complications, too, are risk factors for hearing impairment. Furthermore, infant low birthweight and prematurity have been associated with delayed or aberrant nervous system development as measured by the auditory brainstem response (Salamy, 1984) and cortical auditory evoked potentials (Cone-Wesson, Kurtzberg, & Vaughan, 1987; Kurtzberg, 1989; Kurtzburg, Hilpert, Kreuzer, & Vaughan, 1984).

Cocaine Effects on Human Neurobehavioral Development

Maternal cocaine use affects neurobehavioral development in the offspring. Cocaine exposed human neonates have poor response to and interaction with their environment and difficulty regulating state (Chasnoff, Burns, & Burns, 1987). Electroencephalographic recordings and clinical neurological examinations reveal signs of central nervous system irritability in ICAMs (Doberczak, Shanzer, Senie, & Kandall, 1988). Increased rates of perinatal cerebral infarctions have been documented (Chasnoff, Bussey, Stack, & Savich, 1986; Dixon & Bejar, 1988). Aberrant respiratory patterns in cocaine-exposed infants suggest dysfunction of brainstem reticular formation sites involved in respiratory control (Chasnoff, Hunt, Ketter, & Kaplan, 1989; Ward et al., 1989). Abnormal performance on neonatal behavioral assessment scales are found for ICAMs, even when gestational cocaine exposure is limited to the first trimester (Chasnoff & Griffith, 1989). These findings in the neonatal period suggest that neurologic, cognitive, and behavioral development will be abnormal. There is no reason to suspect that the auditory nervous system would be spared.

Long-term neurobehavioral sequelae for ICAMs are being investigated. These infants may demonstrate deviant psychological behavior related to the psychopharmacology of cocaine (Howard, 1989). Drug-exposed infants tested with the Bayley Scales of Infant Development had lower mental developmental and psychomotor developmental index scores than did normal (nondrug) controls, but scores for most infants were still in the normal range (Chasnoff & Schnoll, 1987). Specific deficits in language development have been shown in a group of infants born to polydrug abusers (Van Barr, 1990).

The neurobehavioral compromise of these infants suggests that commonly used measures of audition based upon behavior, such as behavioral observation or visual reinforcement audiometry, may not be valid, or

reliable. Furthermore, it is difficult to parcel out the long-term neurobehavioral effects of gestational drug exposure from the effects of an early childhood spent in a milieu of poverty and parental drug abuse. Electrophysiologic tests of audition, such as the auditory brainstem response or cortical auditory event-related potentials, may help to define neurodevelopmental effects of maternal cocaine abuse in the sensory system most crucial for oral language development. Electrophysiologic probes offer a means for evaluating the infant at an early age, and thus separate the effects of gestational drug exposure from environmental factors.

Cocaine Effects on Neurobehavioral Development — Animal Models

The concept of "developmental toxicity" (Vorhees, 1989) can be used to define the search for the effects of prenatal cocaine exposure on infant development. Developmental toxicity refers to the postnatal structural or functional effects of prenatal toxic substance exposure. According to Vorhees (1989), two important principles in this field are:

(1) Developmental injuries to the nervous system have a protracted period of susceptability which extends beyond organogenesis.
(2) The most frequent injuries to the developing nervous system do not result in CNS malformations, but rather functional abnormalities. Such effects are often not detectable at birth. (p. 33)

Results from studies utilizing gestationally exposed experimental animals underscore cocaine's developmental toxicity. Rat pups exposed during a critical period of synaptic development show increased motor activity as well as long-term changes in the neuro-chemistry of the dopaminergic system (Dow-Edwards, 1989). The rat model of gestational cocaine exposure reveals that cognitive function is impaired for some memory and learning tasks (Spear, Kirstein, & Frambes, 1989).

These animal studies suggest that the neurodevelopmental effect of cocaine may be expressed during infancy or later, when behavior, learning, and memory can be quantified specifically. On the other hand, the use of electrophysiologic probes of central nervous system development may be sensitive to the neurodevelopmental effects of cocaine.

Acute Effects of Cocaine on Auditory System — Animal Models

Cocaine has a deleterious effect on the auditory nervous system. Jacobson, Bedford, Eisele, and Turner (1985) identified toxic effects of cocaine on the primate auditory system. This group showed that acutely cocaine intoxicated macaque monkeys had abnormal auditory brainstem evoked responses (ABRs) in comparison to the nonintoxicated control state. Similarly, Gritzke and Church (1988) demonstrated that adult rats treated with cocaine had elevated ABR thresholds and an abnormally steep slope for the latency-intensity functions. These cocaine-induced changes were interpreted as evidence of cochlear or cochlear nucleus dysfunction. Both studies demonstrated that cocaine has neuro- and ototoxic effects. These studies were an impetus to study the effects of prenatal cocaine exposure on human newborns.

Current Findings

There was reason to believe that maternal cocaine use could have a deleterious effect on the developing auditory system. Our first study (Shih et al., 1988) used the auditory brainstem response (ABR) to document auditory system status in 18 full-term infants born to cocaine-abusing women and an equal number of full-term (nondrug exposed) control infants.

The first question asked was whether there was any frank hearing impairment among newborn ICAMs. The lowest signal level at which an ABR can be recorded has a high correlation with pure tone threshold in the 2k to 4k Hz frequency range (Gorga, Worthington, Reiland, Beauchaine, & Goldhar, 1985). Long-term followup comparing ABRs recorded in early infancy to pure tone thresholds measured in early childhood demonstrates that this measurement has high sensitivity and specificity for hearing impairment detection (Hyde, Matsumoto, & Alberti, 1990). In the Shih, Cone-Wesson, and Reddix (1988) study, ABRs were tested using signal levels at 20 to 80 dB nHL. They measured ABR peak latencies (interval between signal and response onset) and noted the lowest signal level for ABR detection. These ABR response parameters are used to measure the degree and type of hearing impairment (Galambos & Hecox, 1978; Gorga et al, 1985). There was no evidence of increased hearing impairment among ICAMs compared to control group infants. While there were some infants in both groups that had no response at 20 or 30 dB nHL signal levels, all ICAMs had responses present at 40 dB nHL, and all but one of the normal control infants had an ABR present at this level. It should be noted that 40 dB nHL has been used as a "cut-off" level for screening high-risk infants for hearing impairment (Hyde et al, 1990). Thus, all ICAMs passed this hearing screening level. Also, the distribution of ABR thresholds was equivalent for the ICAM and control groups. Finally, the ABR latency change as a function of signal level was equivalent in the two groups. These findings indicated that peripheral hearing among ICAMS was equivalent to those of normal cohorts. Since this study used signals below 40 dB nHL, even mild impairment, if present, would have been detected. These findings have been replicated in our lab using similar sized samples of full-term (Cone-Wesson, unpublished data) and low birthweight ICAMs (Cone-Wesson & Spingarn, 1990).

The second question asked was whether infant central auditory nervous system function, as measured by ABR, was affected by maternal cocaine use. The ABR Wave I to Wave V interpeak latency (I–V IPL) is a measure of central auditory system function. The latency of ABR Wave I, generated by eighth nerve activity, is subtracted from the latency of ABR Wave V, generated by upper brainstem activity. The latency difference is known also as central transmission time, an indicator of neural conduction in the brainstem (Salamy, 1984). The I–V IPL decreases during the first 18 to 24 months of life (Hecox & Burkhard, 1982), a maturational change related to increased myelination of the brainstem (Salamy, 1984). The I–V IPL has been used to indicate disease or lesion to the brainstem auditory nervous system (Hecox, Cone, & Blaw, 1981; Starr, 1977; Stockard & Rossiter, 1977), neurodevelopmental delay (Salamy, 1984), and correlates with several aspects of neurobehavioral function (Murray, 1988). We suspected that the I–V IPL in ICAMs would be prolonged relative to control group infants, indicating central auditory nervous system dysfunction or neuromaturational delay.

Prolonged Wave I–V IPLs in ICAMs have been found by Shih et al. (1988), Cone-Wesson and Spingarn (1990) and by Salamy et al. (1990). Shih et al. (1988) demonstrated this effect in a sample of full-term ICAMs. Cone-Wesson and Spingarn (1990) extended this finding to low-birth-weight ICAMs compared to low-birthweight control infants. They further showed that this effect was present over a significant range of signal levels and presentation rates used to elicit ABRs. Salamy et al (1990) demonstrated that prolonged I–V IPLs for ICAMs, found at 32 to 44 weeks conceptional age, reached normal values during the first 6 months of life.

Prolonged I–V IPLs suggest that there is abnormal neural transmission time for the cocaine-compromised infant auditory system. Alternately, prolonged interpeak latencies indicate delayed brainstem auditory system development (Salamy, 1984).

Prolonged ABR interpeak latencies for ICAMs may reflect neurotransmitter dysfunction or depletion at the level of the brainstem. In the animal model, cocaine disrupts neurotransmitter function at several nervous system levels, including the brainstem (Dow-Edwards, 1989). Anoxia may also be a significant factor resulting in prolonged ABR latencies. Cocaine causes placenta vasoconstriction, decreasing fetal blood flow and oxygenation (Woods, Plessinger, & Clark, 1987). Prolonged or repeated incidents of anoxia or hypoxia impairs the central nervous system, and the brainstem is particularly sensitive to oxygen deprivation. Prolonged interpeak latencies have been reported in infants compromised by oxygen deprivation (Hecox & Cone, 1981; Kileny, Connely, & Robertson, 1980).

The functional implications of prolonged I–V IPL have not been determined. It is one of several auditory evoked potential abnormalities that have been found in older children with speech and language delays (Mason & Mellor, 1984). Murray (1988) found correlations between neonatal I–V IPL and behavioral responses such as orienting, motor maturity, and state organization. She concluded that the I–V IPL could be a useful indicator of CNS function in high-risk newborns. The prolonged I–V IPL latencies found in the reported studies argue for the existence of subtle differences in brainstem auditory system function in ICAMs, even when peripheral auditory system function is normal (Cone-Wesson & Spingarn, 1990; Shih et al., 1988).

Future Directions

The ototoxic effects of cocaine seen in the animal research have not been found in human infants exposed to cocaine in utero. The infant born at full term with either slightly subnormal or normal birthweight appears to have normal peripheral auditory system sensitivity as measured by ABRs. No increased incidence of hearing impairment has been proven in these ICAMs. The neurotoxic effects of cocaine, on the other hand, appear to be evident in the CANS, where abnormal neural transmission time is evident in ICAM group data. The CANS functional abnormality appears in both full-term and low-birthweight ICAMs when compared to an age- and weight-matched cohort (Cone-Wesson & Spingarn, 1990; Salamy et al., 1990).

The fact remains, however, that many ICAMs are born prematurely, and of low birthweight (Chouteau et al, 1988; MacGregor, Keith, Bachicha, & Chasnoff, 1989). Infants compromised by prematurity and low birthweight are at risk for hearing impairment and other neurologic sequelae (Kitchen, Ford, Rickards, Lissenden, & Ryan, 1987). The incidence of hearing impairment among neonatal intensive care unit graduates (with most graduates being those compromised by extreme prematurity) is estimated at 2 to 5%, 10 to 20 times the incidence in a normal full-term cohort (Carter & Wilkening, 1991). The ICAM samples tested by Cone-Wesson and Spingarn (1990) and Salamy et al. (1990) included some premature very low-birthweight in-fants in both ICAM and control groups. These samples, however, were not large enough to address the question of increased risk of peripheral hearing impairment among ICAM-NICU graduates compared to a NICU-graduate control group. Based upon the data from full-term infants, exposure to cocaine alone does not appear to increase the risk for peripheral hearing impairment. Maternal cocaine use is a risk factor for peripheral hearing impairment insofar as the infant is at risk for premature birth, low birthweight, and the medical complications arising from these conditions.

There are no studies that have used more traditional measures of peripheral sensitivity, such as visual reinforcement audiometry or conditioned play audiometry (Kile & Beauchaine, 1991) to test older infants or children with a history of exposure to cocaine in utero. These infants have been shown to have poor interaction with the environment and may be irritable as well (Chasnoff et al., 1987; Dobserczak et al., 1988). These characteristics could preclude accurate behavioral measures of hearing sensitivity. The ABR, then, would be the preferred test method for these infants and children.

Central auditory system function or maturation appears to be affected by maternal cocaine use. More research is needed to elucidate the functional implications of prolonged ABR Wave I-V IPLs. There has been little research correlating ABR with perceptual measures of central auditory system function. Central auditory system dysfunction is thought to be a factor in some learning disabilities (Keith, 1981). Behavioral tests for central auditory system function rely upon sophisticated signal and response paradigms that are not usually adaptable for testing infants or young children. Thus, we must define the neural substrates of auditory perception and central auditory system function using auditory evoked potential techniques.

This task may be approached by using evoked potential signal paradigms that tap central auditory system function at brainstem and cortical levels. For example, complex auditory skills such as localization or separation of signal from noise, rely upon the comparison of incoming signals from the two ears. For this reason, perceptual tests for central auditory function often rely upon binaural (two ears together) presentation of signals (Tobin, 1985). The difference between monaural (single ear) and binaural signal presentation for eliciting ABRs in normal, ICAM, and other infants at risk for central auditory nervous system dysfunction is currently being investigated by Cone-Wesson and her colleagues at the LAC+USC Medical Center.

Auditory cortex and cortical association areas are needed for interpretation and cognitive elaboration of complex acoustic signals such as speech. Cortical auditory system integrity may be investigated using evoked potential techniques. The middle latency response, the cortical event related potential (Kileny, 1985) and the cortical evoked mismatched negativity response (Nymann et al., 1990) are electrophysiologic responses that may be used to describe cortical auditory system function. Cone-Wesson has undertaken a study of monaural and binaural evoked middle latency responses in normal and ICAM infants designed to detect any differences in cortical activity for these two groups. The hypothesis is that ICAMs, who have demonstrated central auditory system abnormality at brainstem level, may also show dysfunction or abnormality at the cortical level of auditory nervous system processing.

Implications For Intervention

It will be difficult to initiate intervention until specific cognitive or perceptual disabilities can be directly related to auditory evoked potential abnormalities. The power of the auditory evoked potential tests is that they can be used to test for peripheral hearing impairment that might otherwise go undetected and untreated. Since many ICAMs will meet one or more risk criteria for hearing impairment, it is imperative that guidelines for hearing screening (Joint Committee on Infant Hearing, 1991) and assessment (ASHA, 1991) be followed.

The risk for neurodevelopmental problems is underscored by the finding of brainstem auditory system neural transmission delays for cocaine-exposed neonates. Neurodevelopmental insult caused by cocaine suggests that these infants should be targeted for speech, language, and cognitive assessment at the earliest possible time. Intervention should be structured from these evaluations.

Acknowledgment

Daniel Kempler provided a helpful critique of an earlier version of this manuscript.

References

ASHA Committee on Infant Hearing. (1991). Guidelines for the audiometric assessment of children from birth through 36 months. *ASHA 33*, (Suppl. 5), 37–43.

Bingol, N., Fuchs, M., Diaz, V., Stone, R. K., & Gromish, D. S. (1987). Teratogenicity of cocaine in humans. *Journal of Pediatrics, 110*, 93–96.

Carter, B. S. & Wilkening, R. B. (1991). Prevention of hearing disorders: Neonatal causes of hearing loss. *Seminars in Hearing, 12*, 154–167.

Chasnoff, I. J., Burns, K. A., & Burns, W. J. (1987). Cocaine use in pregnancy: Perinatal morbidity and mortality. *Neurotoxicology and Teratology, 9*, 291–293.

Chasnoff, I. J., Burns, W. J., Schnoll, S. H., & Burns, K. A. (1985). Cocaine use in pregnancy. *New England Journal of Medicine, 313,* 666–669.

Chasnoff, I. J., Bussey, M. E., Stack, C. A., & Savich, R. (1986). Perinatal cerebral infarction and maternal cocaine use. *Journal of Pediatrics, 108,* 456–459.

Chasnoff, I. J., Chisum, G. M., & Kaplan, W. E. (1988). Maternal cocaine use and genitourinary tract malformations. *Teratology, 37,* 201–204.

Chasnoff, I. J., & Griffith, D. R. (1989). Cocaine: Clinical studies of pregnancy and the newborn. *Annals of the New York Academy of Sciences, 562,* 260–266.

Chasnoff, I. J., Hunt, C. E., Ketter, R., & Kaplan, D. (1989). Prenatal cocaine exposure is associated with respiratory pattern abnormalities. *American Journal of Disorders of Childhood, 143,* 583–587.

Chasnoff, I. J., & Schnoll, S. H. (1987). Consequences of cocaine and other drug use in pregnancy. In A. M. Washton & M. S. Gold (Eds.). *Cocaine. A clinician's handbook.* (pp 241–251). New York: The Guilford Press.

Chouteau, M., Namerow, P. B., & Leppert, P. (1988). The effect of cocaine abuse on birthweight and gestational age. *Obstetrics and Gynecology, 72,* 351–354.

Clarren, S. K., & Smith, D. W. (1978). The fetal alcohol syndrome: Experience with 65 patients and a review of the world literature. *New England Journal of Medicine, 298,* 1065–1067.

Cone-Wesson, B., Kurtzberg, D., & Vaughan, H. G. (1987). Electrophysiologic assessment of auditory pathways in high risk infants. *International Journal of Pediatric Otorhinolaryngology, 14,* 203–214.

Cone-Wesson, B., & Spingarn, A. (1990). Effects of maternal cocaine abuse on neonatal ABR: Premature and small-for-dates infants. *Journal of the American Academy of Audiology, 1,* 52(A).

Dixon, S. D., & Bejar, R. (1988). Brain lesions in cocaine and methamphetamine-exposed neonates. *Pediatric Research, 23,* 405(A).

Doberczak, T. M., Shanzer, S., Senie, R. T., & Kandall, S. R. (1988). Neonatal neurologic and electroencephalic effects of intrauterine cocaine exposure. *Journal of Pediatrics, 113,* 354–358.

Dow-Edwards, D. L. (1989). Long-term neurochemical and neurobehavioral consequences of cocaine use during pregnancy. *Annals of the New York Academy of Sciences, 562,* 280–289.

Galambos, R. & Hecox, K. E. (1978). Clinical applications of the auditory brainstem response. *Otolaryngology Clinics of North America, 11* 709–722.

Gorga, M., Worthington, D., Reiland, J., Beauchaine, K., & Goldhar, D. (1985). Some comparisons between auditory brainstem response thresholds, latencies and the pure tone audiogram. *Ear and Hearing, 6,* 105–112.

Gritzke, R. & Church, M. W. (1988). Effects of cocaine on the brainstem auditory evoked potential in the Long-Evans rat. *Electroencephalography and Clinical Neurophysiology, 71,* 389–399.

Hecox, K. E. & Burkhard, R. (1982). Developmental dependencies of the human brainstem auditory evoked responses. *Annals of the New York Academy of Sciences, 388,* 538–556.

Hecox, K. E., Cone, B., & Blaw, M. (1981). Brainstem auditory evoked response in the diagnosis of pediatric neurologic diseases. *Neurology, 31,* 829–839.

Hecox, K. E. & Cone, B. K. (1981). Prognostic importance of brainstem auditory evoked response after asphyxia. *Neurology, 31,* 1429–1433.

Howard, J. (1989). Cocaine and its effects on the newborn. *Developmental Medicine and Child Neurology, 31,* 255–263.

Hoyme, H. E., Jones, K. L., Dixon, S. D., Dixon, S. D., Jewett, T., Hanson, J. W., Robinson, L. K., Msall, M. E., & Allanson, J. E. (1990). Prenatal cocaine exposure and fetal vascular disruption. *Pediatrics, 85,* 743–747.

Hyde, M. L., Matsumoto, N., & Alberti, P. W. (1990). Audiometric accuracy of the click ABR in infants at risk for hearing loss. *Journal of the American Academy of Audiology, 1,* 59–66.

Jacobson, J. T., Bedford, J. A., Eisele, W. A., & Turner, B. (1985). Effects of delta-9 THC and cocaine on ABR in monkeys. *ASHA, 27,* 182(A).

Joint Committee on Infant Hearing. (1991). Position statement. *American Academy of Otolaryngology — Head and Neck Surgery Bulletin,* March, 15-18.

Keith, R. W. (1981). Tests of central auditory function. In R. J. Roeser & M. P. Downs (Eds.), *Auditory disorders in school children* (pp. 159-173). New York: Thieme-Stratton.

Kile, J. E., & Beauchaine, K. L. (1991). Identification, assessment, and management of hearing impairment in infants and toddlers. *Infant-Toddler Intervention, 1,* 62-81.

Kileny, P. (1985). Middle latency (MLR) and late vertex auditory evoked responses (LVAER) in central auditory dysfunction. In M. L. Pinheiro & F. E. Musiek (Eds.)., *Assessment of central auditory dysfunction. Foundations and clinical correlates* (pp. 87-102). New York: Williams and Wilkins.

Kileny, P., Connely, C., & Robertson, C. (1980). Auditory brainstem responses in perinatal asphyxia. *International Journal of Pediatric Otorhinolaryngology, 2,* 147-159.

Kitchen, W. H., Ford, G. W., Rickards, A. L., Lissenden, J. V., & Ryan, M. R. (1987). Children of birthweight < 1000 g.: Changing outcome between ages 2 and 5 years. *Journal of Pediatrics, 110,* 283-288.

Kurtzberg, D. (1989). Cortical event-related potential assessment of auditory system function. *Seminars in Hearing, 10,* 252-261.

Kurtzberg, D., Hilpert, P. L., Kreuzer, J. A., & Vaughan, H. G. (1984). Differential maturation of cortical auditory evoked potentials to speech sounds in normal full-term and very low-birthweight infants. *Developmental Medicine and Child Neurology, 26,* 466-475.

Little, B. B., Snell, L. M., Palmore, M. K., & Gilstrap, L. C. (1988). Cocaine use in pregnant women in a large public hospital. *American Journal of Perinatology, 5,* 206-207.

MacGregor, S. N., Keith, L. G., Bachicha, J. A., & Chasnoff, I. J. (1989). Cocaine abuse during pregnancy: Correlation between prenatal care and perinatal outcome. *Obstetrics and Gynecology, 74,* 882-885.

Mason, B. M., & Mellor, D. H. (1984). Brainstem, middle latency and late cortical evoked potentials in children with speech and language disorders. *Electroencephalography and Clinical Neurophysiology, 59,* 297-309.

Møller, A. B., Jannetta, P. J., & Møller, M. B. (1981). Neural generators of the brainstem evoked responses: Results from human intracranial recordings. *Annals of Otology, Rhinology and Laryngology, 90,* 591-596.

Murray, A. D. (1988). Newborn auditory brainstem evoked responses (ABRs): Prenatal and contemporary correlates. *Child Development, 59,* 571-588.

Nyman, G., Alho, K., Laurinen, P., Paavilainen, P., Radil, R., Reinikainen, K., Sams, M., & Naatanen, R. (1990). Mismatch negativity (MMN) for sequences of auditory and visual stimuli: Evidence for a mechanism specific to the auditory modality. *Electroencephalography and Clinical Neurophysiology, 77,* 151-155.

Oro, A. S., Dixon, S. D. (1987). Perinatal cocaine and methamphetamine exposure: Maternal and neonatal correlates. *Journal of Pediatrics, 111,* 571-578.

Picton, T. W., Taylor, M. J., Durieux-Smith, A., & Edwards, C. G. (1986). Brainstem auditory evoked potentials in pediatrics. In M. J. Aminoff (Ed.), *Electrodiagnosis in clinical neurology* (pp. 505-534). New York: Churchill Livingstone.

Rottveel, J. J., Colon, E. J., Stegman, D. F., & Visco, Y. M. (1987a). The maturation of the central auditory conduction in preterm infants until three months post-term. I. Composite group averages of brainstem (ABR) and middle latency (MLR) auditory evoked responses. *Hearing Research, 26,* 11-20.

Rottveel, J. J., deGraf, R., Colon, E. J., Stegman, D. F., & Visco, Y. M. (1987b). The maturation of the central auditory conduction in pre-term infants until three months post-term. II. The auditory brainstem responses (ABR). *Hearing Research, 26,* 21-35.

Ryan, L., Ehrlich, S., & Finnegan, L. P. (1987). Cocaine abuse in pregnancy: Effects on the fetus and newborn. *Neurotoxicology and Teratology, 9,* 295-299.

Salamy, A. (1984). Maturation of the auditory

brainstem response from birth through early childhood. *Journal of Clinical Neurophysiology, 1,* 293–329.

Salamy, A., Eldredge, L., Anderson, J., & Bull, D. (1990). Brainstem transmission time in infants exposed to cocaine in utero. *Journal of Pediatrics, 117,* 627–629.

Shih, L., Cone-Wesson, B., & Reddix, B. (1988). Effects of maternal cocaine abuse on the neonatal auditory system. *International Journal of Pediatric Otorhinolaryngology, 15,* 245–251.

Spear, L. P., Kirstein, D. L., & Frambes, N. A. (1989). Cocaine effects on the developing central nervous system: Behavioral, psychopharmacological and neurochemical studies. *Annals of the New York Academy of Sciences, 562,* 290–307.

Starr, A. (1977). Clinical relevance of brainstem auditory evoked potentials in brainstem disorders in man. In J. E. Desmedt (Ed.), *Auditory evoked potentials in man: Vol. 2. Psychopharmacology correlates of evoked potentials* (pp. 45–57). Basel: Karger.

Stockard, J. J. & Rossiter, V. G. (1977). Clinical and pathologic correlates of brainstem auditory response abnormalities. *Neurology, 27,* 316–325.

Tobin, H. (1985). Binaural interaction tasks. In M. L. Pinheiro & F. E. Musiek (Eds.), *Assessment of central auditory dysfunction. Foundations and clinical correlates* (pp. 155–171). New York: Williams and Wilkins.

Van Baar, A. (1990). Development of infants of drug-dependent mothers. *Journal of Child Psychology and Psychiatry, 31,* 911–920.

Vorhees, C. V. (1989). Concepts in teratology and developmental toxicology derived from animal research. *Annals of the New York Academy of Sciences, 562,* 31–41.

Ward, S. L. D., Bautista, D. B., Schuetz, S., Wachsman, L., Bean, X., & Keens, T. G. (1989). Abnormal hypoxic arousal responses in infants of cocaine-abusing mothers. *Annals of the New York Academy of Sciences, 562,* 347–348.

Woods, J. R., Plessinger, M. A., & Clark, K. E. (1987). Effect of cocaine use on uterine blood flow and fetal oxygenation. *Journal of the American Medical Association, 257,* 957–961.

Address correspondence to:
Barbara Cone-Wesson, Ph.D.,
Audiology Clinic
LAC+USC Medical Center
Outpatient Department, #2P70
1175 Cummings Street
Los Angeles, CA 90033

Prenatal Cocaine Exposure: The Challenge to Education

Sharon Lesar, M.Ed.

University of California, Santa Barbara

Research in the past 10 years has produced a growing amount of new literature and speculations about the effects on infants who have been exposed to cocaine in utero. Concern over the expanding number of women cocaine abusers has led to increased attention on identifying the problems and needs of children exposed to cocaine in utero, because it is one aspect of a complex set of problems that influences the child's development. The risk factors associated with prenatal cocaine exposure are particularly relevant in light of P.L. 99-457. This article discusses the impact of maternal cocaine use during pregnancy, early intervention recommendations, the impact on professionals, areas of research, and the challenge to education as the magnitude of the problem increases.

Over the past decade, a major concern has emerged regarding the effects of prenatal exposure to illegal drugs, especially cocaine. With the increasing use of cocaine in the United States, there has been growing concern regarding its effects on the fetuses and neonates of pregnant cocaine abusers (Chasnoff, Burns, & Burns, 1987). In addition to causing problems before birth and in the newborn and infancy period, it is feared that prenatal drug abuse may cause long-term effects during childhood, such as behavior disorders and learning disabilities. As this generation of children, whose mothers abused drugs, approach school age, a number of unique issues have surfaced. Questions regarding the impact of drugs on children, mothers, and the helping professionals, the types of intervention required, and

clinical and treatment issues are being addressed by researchers (Chasnoff, 1988; Pawl, 1989). If we are to understand fully the development of children exposed to cocaine in utero, specific environment risk factors, such as maternal characteristics, degrees of life stress, patterns of child-care, and the qualitative characteristics of mother-child interactions also must be examined. It may well be that prenatal exposure to cocaine is only a symptom of other facets of lifestyle and environment that must be addressed if a child is to reach his or her full potential.

Hospitals in major cities throughout the country are reporting escalating numbers of infants being born to mothers who use cocaine. In a hospital survey conducted by the Select Committee on Children, Youth and

Infant-Toddler Intervention.
The Transdisciplinary Journal (Vol. 2, No. 1, pp. 37–52)
© 1992, Singular Publishing Group, Inc.

Families (Miller, 1989), 15 of the 18 hospitals reported that since 1980 cocaine has become the drug of choice for pregnant women at an exceedingly high rate, penetrating all socioeconomic lines. In a Houston hospital, the percentage of pregnant substance abusers reporting cocaine use increased from 2% in 1980 to more than 80% in 1989. In San Francisco County Hospital, 16% of the children born at that hospital were born to cocaine-addicted mothers (American Academy of Pediatrics, 1988), and a hospital in Philadelphia reports the number of drug-exposed newborns rose from 4% in 1987 to 15% in 1988, based on newborn toxic screening and maternal histories (Miller, 1989). These numbers appear to be similar for hospitals outside larger urban areas. For example, a hospital in Ft. Lauderdale, Florida, reported that 20% of the infants tested positive for cocaine in 1987, and a suburban area in California reported 40 babies a month were born drug-exposed (Miller, 1989).

Currently, "crack" is the most commonly used form of cocaine. Crack is a highly concentrated form of cocaine; however, the effect is relatively brief, resulting in repeated uses of the drug which can create a pattern that can lead to high levels of fetal exposure in pregnant women (Smith, 1988). However, crack is seldom used alone. To cloud the picture further, cocaine users often use other illegal substances such as alcohol, marijuana, and tranquilizers. This multi-drug use has an even greater negative impact on the mother and her fetus (Kronstadt, 1989).

Effects of Cocaine

Effects on the Fetus and Newborn

Cocaine use during pregnancy has been associated with having significant effects on pregnancy and the developing fetus (Chasnoff, Burns, & Burns, 1987; Schneider & Chasnoff, 1987; Schneider, Griffith, & Chasnoff, 1989; Smith, 1988). Some obstetrical complications found in drug-dependent women include abruptio placentae, in utero cerebrovascular accidents, spontaneous abortions, toxemia, retained placenta, postpartum hemorrhage, and premature delivery (Finnegan, 1976). Table 1 lists some of the obstetrical complications encountered in cocaine addicts. In addition, among drug-addicted women who are prostitutes, infections such as syphilis and those of the urinary tract are found during pregnancy. Needles used by pregnant women can cause other complications such as hepatitis B, venous thrombosis, abscesses (Finnegan, 1976), and acquired immunodeficiency syndrome (AIDS). Lack of adequate diet may contribute to anemia, vitamin deficiencies, and malnutrition of the fetus, since cocaine has an anorexic effect and causes the user to have a decreased interest in bodily needs (Ryan, Ehrlich, & Finnegan, 1987). Women cocaine users who do not enter treatment

Table 1. Obstetrical complications of addicted women

Abortion
Abruptio placentae
Amnionitis
Breech presentation
Previous C-section
Chorioamnionitis
Eclampsia
Gestational diabetes
Intrauterine death
Intrauterine growth retardation
Placental insufficiency
Post-partum hemorrhage
Pre-eclampsia
Preterm labor
Premature rupture of membranes
Septic thrombophlebitis

for their addiction, either before or during pregnancy, may receive little or no prenatal care, thus increasing the probability of complications during delivery, and the likelihood of problems for the fetus.

Cocaine neonates do not go through the intense drug withdrawal documented in infants born to heroin-addicted mothers; however, controversy exists over the presence of a cocaine withdrawal syndrome. Within this group of cocaine-exposed infants is a spectrum of outcomes, ranging from those with no observable effects to those in great distress immediately after birth. Some of the identified symptoms of this withdrawal include irritability, overexcitability, poor feeding patterns, high respiratory and heart rates, increased tremulousness and startles, and unusually stiff muscles. These infants can display a high-pitched cry and are very sensitive to the mildest environmental stimulation. They may not fall asleep readily, and once asleep, are easily awakened. The distress of these newborns is obvious, and yet they are unable to calm themselves (Schneider & Chasnoff, 1987; Schneider, Griffith, & Chasnoff, 1989; Smith, 1988). Even though these infants may be in distress, other possibilities or mechanisms that could cause physiologic and behavioral outcomes, such as acute toxicity, must be taken into account. Many of the outcomes of cocaine exposure are difficult to tease apart from other confounding risk factors; for example, low socioeconomic status, low birthweight, premature birth, and so forth. However, maternal cocaine use adds a potential biological insult that may increase the child's vulnerability over and above all other factors.

In contrast, some cocaine-exposed infants may experience the opposite characteristics. Cocaine-exposed newborns may retreat into a deep sleep in an attempt to eliminate all environmental stimulation, and they may sleep much of the time. In addi-tion, they are unresponsive to the overtures of their caregivers (Kronstadt, 1989).

Chasnoff, Burns, Schnoll, and Burns (1985) found that when tested using the Brazelton Neonatal Behavioral Assessment Scale infants exposed to cocaine had significant depression of interactive behavior and a poor organizational response to environmental stimuli (state organization). These physiologic and behavioral findings suggest that cocaine exposure in utero interferes with an infant's ability to maintain adequate state control in the neonatal period. Not only did these infants display poor state control and poor interactive abilities when compared to a nondrug-exposed group, but the cocaine-exposed group also showed significant differences in many reflex and motor responses. Compared to the methadone, multi-drug, and drug-free groups, the cocaine-addicted newborns obtained poorer consolability scores as a group. The cocaine-exposed infants needed maximum intervention from the examiner to achieve even partial calming. Findings from this project document that infants from all drug-exposed groups exhibited compromised developmental status as neonates, but infants born to cocaine-abusing women were the most compromised of infants during the neonatal period. This factor places these infants in a category of high risk because initially they may be incapable of responding appropriately to their caregivers.

Studies have shown that the behavior of the newborn affects the caregiving he or she receives (Osofsky, 1976; Osofsky & Danrger, 1974). The reciprocity normally present in the bonding process may not be established because of the behavior of the poorly organized, high-risk infant. In effect, a negative cycle may be established in which the infant may suppress the optimal caregiving pattern necessary to facilitate his or her recovery (Schneider & Chasnoff, 1987).

The state control dimension refers to the infant's ability to move appropriately through the various states of arousal in response to the demands of the environment. The well-organized, fully functioning infant will move through each of the states of arousal that is appropriate for the level and type of stimulation the infant is encountering, and the transition will be relatively smooth from state to state. However, many cocaine-exposed infants are rarely well-organized, fully functioning infants. Instead they spend most of their time in states that shut them off from external stimulation, and their state changes tend to be abrupt and inappropriate for the level of stimulation encountered (Griffith, 1988).

Griffith (1988) reported data on the state control abilities of cocaine-exposed infants at 1 month of age, as measured by the Neonatal Behavioral Assessment Scale (NBAS). Most of these infants were capable of reaching all of the various states of arousal; however, many still have very low thresholds for overstimulation. These infants required a great deal of careful handling and containment from the examiner to reach and/or maintain responsive states. Without examiner assistance, they often display abrupt, inappropriate state changes in response to the demands of the exam. Even with the assistance provided by the examiner, there were a few 1-month-old, cocaine-exposed infants who seemed unable to tolerate even low levels of stimulation. These infants vacillated quickly from an agitated cry state in response to most types of stimulation to a deep-sleep state in which they shut themselves off from all external stimulation. Even the soothing techniques of the examiner did not assist the infant. Only by pulling down into a deep sleep, or by displaying a self-perpetuating and long-lasting cry state are they able to shut out external stimulation.

Another area of difficulty for the cocaine-exposed infant is orientation. Orientation refers to the infant's ability to interact actively with the outside world by attending to and responding to visual and auditory stimuli, presented either singly or simultaneously (Griffith, 1988). The well-organized, normal, drug-free newborn typically can achieve repeated episodes of responsiveness to external stimuli with varying degrees of examiner assistance. By 1 month of age, they are able to respond appropriately to visual and auditory stimuli for lengthy periods of time with little or no assistance from the examiner. In contrast, the orientation abilities of newborn cocaine-exposed infants are quite limited. Many of these infants are unable to reach an alert responsive state. Even using containment techniques to induce an alert state, such as tight swaddling, use of a pacifier, hand holding, and vertical rocking, most newborn, cocaine-exposed infants are capable of only fleeting attention to a stimulus before showing signs of distress. In addition, each stimulus presented seems to have a cumulative effect toward overloading the infants, so that the infants are less responsive to each successive stimulus. Once the level of stimulation is too great, these infants either go into a sleep state, or move into an unavailable crying state.

Some additional effects of cocaine on infants prenatally exposed to it throughout pregnancy include a decrease in mean birthweight, length, head circumference, and Apgar scores (Ryan, Ehrlich, & Finnegan, 1987). These researchers describe three groups of subjects, consisting of 50 women each, who either used cocaine, were maintained on methadone with no cocaine use, or were nondrug-dependent women. Their findings suggest that parameters defining fetal and infant outcome are poorer when the mother is drug dependent during pregnancy, and that cocaine-exposed infants have even poorer outcomes.

In addition, the cocaine group's fetal death rate is twice that of noncocaine, drug-dependent women, and infants exposed to cocaine have a greater incidence of sudden infant death syndrome (SIDS). The rate of SIDS in cocaine-exposed infants may be as high as 15%, more than three times the rate in heroin-exposed infants (Smith, 1988).

In another study investigating the effects of cocaine on pregnancy and the neonate, Chasnoff (1988) reports similar information. During a 10-year period, 75 infants born to cocaine-using women were compared to a drug-free comparison group of 70 infants with similar social, demographic, and environmental backgrounds. Chasnoff reports an increase in complications of labor and delivery and an increased incidence of premature labor in cocaine-using women, as compared to drug-free women. The cocaine group of infants had a reduced mean gestational age. When the premature infants were eliminated from the analysis, there was a statistically significant difference in birthweights, lengths, and head circumferences between infants in the two comparison groups.

Caring for the Young Infant of a Cocaine-Addicted Mother

The difficulty in caring for the young infant of a cocaine-addicted mother continues after the neonatal period. The majority of cocaine-exposed infants could be classified as "fragile" infants, with very low thresholds for overstimulation. These infants require a great deal of assistance from caregivers, even experienced ones, to maintain control of their hyperexcitable nervous systems (Chasnoff, 1988). Moreover, their tendency to exhibit irritability, sleep problems, difficulty with calming, and state control place additional stress on the developing mother-infant attachment.

As noted earlier, many cocaine-exposed infants are very irritable, cry more frequently, and are difficult to cuddle. When these infants are paired with cocaine-abusing mothers, it is not surprising that a number of pathological maternal-infant relationships develop. Substance abuse undermines normal patterns of interaction and alters conventional priorities (Howard, Beckwith, Rodning, & Kropenske, 1989). These families often come from a history of impoverishment, abuse, and intergenerational chemical dependence. Many of the women are single, divorced or separated, and have inadequate social supports. Parents who are addicted to drugs have a primary commitment to chemicals, not to their children. Thus, against this backdrop of a disruptive and chaotic environment, low self-esteem, inadequate parenting models, and lack of social support, a newborn with special needs and problems is added, making the situation difficult to manage, even for the best equipped mother.

According to Griffith (1988), many of the cocaine-abusing mothers experience the same feelings about parenthood, and demonstrate the same deficiencies in knowledge that have been seen in other programs treating drug-addicted mothers. These feelings and behaviors range from guilt concerning the potential damage their cocaine abuse may have done to their infant, fearfulness concerning their ability to cope with and successfully meet the demands of their child, and unrealistic expectations about their infant's competencies with respect to normal child development. Many of these mothers appear to detach themselves almost completely from their infants. It has been reported (Griffith, 1988; Howard, Beckwith, Rodning, & Kropenske, 1989) that many of these mothers fail to appear for clinical appointments or follow through on community, health, and social service referrals. When mothers did show up for their appointments, they appeared very lethargic and displayed flat affects. Some substance-abusing mothers had difficulty remembering simple instructions, or exhibited difficulties with attention and perception. During the developmental assessments of their infants, the detached mothers failed to attend to either their infants' behavior, or the feedback provided to them concerning how to better care for their infants. Some mothers often stared blankly at the wall or fell asleep.

The conditions observed in cocaine-exposed infants make these infants very difficult to cuddle and comfort, which has the effect of interrupting the normal processes of maternal/infant attachment that are so important to the early relationship between infant and mother. These behavioral risks identified at birth or during the first month of life have repercussions for later development, inasmuch as infants who have deficits in their ability to maintain a steady state, respond properly to human stimulation, and use proper motor control do not respond appropriately to caretaker initiatives to interact. Consequently, a vicious cycle of infant passivity and maternal rejection is instituted.

In addition to the abnormal behavioral states and interactional behaviors of infants of cocaine-abusing mothers, other factors may be included in the causal chain that produces a dysfunctional mother-infant bond. These factors may include the ineptness of the mother, lack of personal resources for the parent, low socioeconomic status, and maternal personality deviances which lead to poor choices of lifestyle (Burns, 1986). In most cases, women who abuse cocaine during pregnancy are not temporarily experimenting with drugs, but have an enduring, pathological dependence. Addiction or dependency is believed to be a disease. If cocaine abuse is part of their maladaptive lifestyle, then their personality disorder places these mothers at high risk for associated problems such as depression, personality disturbances, and mood and character disturbances. In the Northwestern Memorial Hospital sample of substance-abusing mothers, significant mood disturbances were found through the use of self-report measures such as the Beck Depression Scale (Burns, Melamed, Burns, Chasnoff, & Hatcher, 1986). Many of these mothers interpreted their infants' attempts to shut out external stimulation as personal rejections of them. This perceived rejection may serve to confirm that they are bad mothers, thereby increasing any feelings of depression and worthlessness that these women might be experiencing. Other mothers seem to blame the baby for rejecting them, which can lead to hostile feelings toward the infant and the mother's failure to provide proper care for the specialized needs of her infant during withdrawal. These factors then become part of the causal chain in the production of the mother-infant relationship.

In summary, the effects of perinatal cocaine exposure on the early mother-infant interaction too often is detrimental to the maternal-infant relationship. Any single factor taken by itself is insufficient to produce the intensity of problems associated with the outcome of the mother-child relationship. Rather, it is the cumulative effect of a poor start on the mother-infant interaction, a poor start on environmental supports for proper cognitive and emotional development, a poor start on self-monitoring of state control, and whatever other factors may be involved. Because so many of these factors coincide in families of cocaine abusers, the efforts aimed at improving the maternal-infant relationship, including maternal psychopathology and personality, need to take into account not only aspects of the maternal-infant relationship, but environmental factors as well.

The Impact on Toddlers

The effects of cocaine exposure do not end in infancy. As cocaine-exposed infants enter the toddler period (age 12 to 30 months), the drug-related birth defects may contribute to major developmental difficulties. Howard, Beckwith, Rodning, and Kropenske (1989) compared a group of premature infants born to a sample of women who most commonly had used cocaine during pregnancy, to nondrug-exposed premature infants from similar environments. Even at the age of 18 months, after receiving good medical care and educational therapy, the cocaine-exposed children showed significant differences. They tended to hit their toys or throw them around the room, without apparent motive or provocation. The drug-exposed toddlers had fewer play sequences than the comparison group in a free play setting. They had more impulsive, less goal-directed behavior, and were more prone to temper tantrums. The drug-exposed toddlers were less securely attached to their caregivers than the comparison group.

Chasnoff and Griffith (1989) found similar behaviors in a study of approximately 200 cocaine-exposed infants. Preliminary results from the toddler period include the following descriptions of behavior: "easily frustrated;" "distractible;" "prone to temper tantrums;" "much throwing and banging;" and "difficulty with processing information." Other risk factors in cocaine-exposed toddlers and young children are poor attachment/sense of self and poor organization of behavior (Poulsen, 1989). In summary, these cocaine-exposed children suffer a range of problems, including developmental delay, slow language use, insecurity, bonding difficulties, memory problems, hyperactivity, and severe emotional and behavioral disturbances.

Early Intervention
Prior to Birth

Most experts in the area of early intervention strongly feel that pregnancy affords a window of opportunity for effective intervention with the mother. In a study conducted at the Perinatal Center for Chemical Dependence (Chasnoff, 1988), it was found that cessation of cocaine early in pregnancy reduced the risks of prematurity and intrauterine growth retardation. Thus, the earlier the mother ceases drug use during pregnancy, the better the long-term outcome for the infant. The developmental risks imposed by the maternal use of cocaine are preventable. However, prevention of the problem requires recognition of the hazards that cocaine presents to the pregnant woman and her unborn child. Appropriate intervention for women who are using cocaine when they become pregnant must rely on comprehensive information obtained by health care professionals during prenatal examinations.

The first step in addressing the cocaine epidemic is educating the public and professional sectors about the hazards of cocaine use. Health care agencies and physicians need to be encouraged to identify and refer pregnant women with drug abuse problems for prenatal services and treatment. As more health care professionals identify this high risk population, treatment programs serving the increasing number of drug-using pregnant women and their children need to be developed. Unfortunately, many drug facilities exclude pregnant women. In one recent study in New York City, 54% would not let these mothers in, and those that did had a waiting list of 3 to 6 months (Kantrowitz, Wingert, De La Pena, Gordon, & Padgett, 1990).

Treatment experts strongly recommend that pregnant women be able to leave their provocative living environments where co-caine is readily available and commonly used. Options should include residential treatment programs and/or drug-free hous-ing, including full-time or part-time resi-dence of children. In addition, comprehen-sive outpatient treatment programs for women who are pregnant and/or have chil-dren need to be developed.

In general, all of the intervention pro-grams serving pregnant drug-addicted wo-men and their children should be compre-hensive and provide collaborative and coor-dinated services. This means that programs make available in central sites health care services, family planning, parenting educa-tion, psychosocial supports, job training, substance abuse, counseling, nutritional counseling, respite care, early intervention, transportation, and other essential services. To coordinate all of the treatment needs for drug-exposed infants and their care pro-viders, a case management system must be established.

Infancy

Cocaine-exposed infants with contribut-ing infant and family risk factors should be eligible for early intervention services. Early intervention should include developmen-tal/behavioral monitoring and family fo-cused assessment procedures that evaluate behavioral, affective, motor language, at-tachment, and social problems beginning in infancy. Eligibility criteria for early interven-tion services should not label the infant as handicapped, delayed, or drug-exposed, but instead include them in the larger "at-risk" category to obtain services.

The overall goal of the newborn phase is to increase periods of alertness so that ap-propriate infant-caregiver interactions can occur (Schneider, Griffith, & Chasnoff, 1989). This broad goal can be accomplished by meeting each of the subgoals listed in

Table 2. Infants born to mothers who use co-caine during pregnancy may have multiple medical problems. If they are premature, they may have difficulties related to this state and require appropriate interventions. For example, warning symptoms of over-stimulation such as yawning, hiccoughing, drooping face, and so on need to be watched for and stimulation decreased. These symp-toms also are utilized as warning signs for the cocaine-exposed, full-term infant. For some infants, vestibular stimulation such as rocking, helps to calm them down. For others, swaddling, decreased handling, and soothing techniques may be useful. The use of these techniques will increase the infant's state control and interactive abilities, so that the bonding process between the infant and caregiver can be established.

The overall intervention goal for the in-fancy period is to improve movement pat-terns to enhance interaction and explora-tion. Evaluation of motor development of cocaine-exposed infants at 4 months of age suggests that they have difficulty moving against the forces of gravity, and they dis-play more immature movement patterns than nondrug-exposed infants (Schneider, 1988). As previously discussed, symptoms of the withdrawal syndrome (e.g., increased extensor tone, tremors, and delayed inte-gration of primitive reflexes) continue dur-ing early infancy. In general, cocaine-exposed infants tend to fall more often into the ques-tionable and abnormal range for motor de-velopment than age-matched normal infants.

Evaluating the infant's motor abilities pro-vides many opportunities for early interven-tion. Physical therapy motor assessment provides valuable information about the ef-fects of in utero cocaine exposure on motor development in infancy. Equally important to the developmental assessment is the par-ent education that occurs during the evalua-tion session. Parent education enhances normal infant development and fosters a

Table 2. Summary of Intervention Goals and Management Related to Period of Development

Period of Development	Intervention Goals	Management
Newborn	Increase periods of alertness and interaction	
	Prevent hyperextended posture	Positioning in sidelying
	Decrease irritability, tremors, and overshooting	Swaddling and rocking
		Hydrotherapy graded auditory and visual stimuli
	Improve feeding patterns	Positioning and handling
	Improve feeding posture	
	Decrease facial and oral hypersensitivity	Tactile stimulation to facial and oral areas
	Improve parent handling	Observe Brazelton Model for appropriate behavior
		Demonstrate and return demonstration of appropriate handling
Infancy	Improve movement patterns to enhance interaction and exploration	
	Decrease extensor tone	Supine flexion with lower extremity rotation
		Prevent extensor thrusting in sitting and standing
		Discourage supported standing
		Discourage use of jumpers and walkers
		Carry inflexed position
		Slow, gentle movement through space
	Increase antigravity strength	Prone positioning
		Pivoting in prone position
		Sitting with support for short periods
	Improve parent handling	Demonstrations and return demonstrations of appropriate play and carrying positions and handling techniques

strong parent-infant relationship. Intervention is possible through both direct and indirect parent education concerning their infant's developmental progress. During the physical therapy sessions, the parent/caregiver can observe and participate in the session. As the therapist handles the child during the session, the parent can oberve appropriate ways to deal with their child physically. Parent education, which includes appropriate play, carrying, and handling techniques, changes according to the infant's needs. In addition, the therapist can highlight strengths and weaknesses that their child possesses. By pointing out a new skill that the child has learned, parent-child relationships are reinforced. On the other hand, weaknesses also are pointed out to the parents to explain how these abnormal signs might interfere with normal activities. Weekly or monthly sessions may be necessary to demonstrate developmentally appropriate activities, to teach parents new handling skills, and to confirm to parents their level of skill and understanding.

Preschool and Older Children

Early intervention beyond infancy may be required by many cocaine-exposed children as they begin to appear in worrisome numbers in preschool and elementary classrooms. So far, there are only a handful of programs dedicated to helping drug-exposed children. One such experimental program is in its third year at the Los Angeles Unified School District. The children in this program were identified at birth as drug-exposed. The goal of the program is to provide these children with early intervention during the preschool years so that the majority of them can transition to regular classrooms. These children are placed in small, rigidly structured classes with a teacher and two assistants. The school also has a pediatrician, psychologists, social workers,

and speech and language specialists on staff. These professionals meet weekly with the teachers and the children's caregivers to help with the problems caused not only by the mothers' cocaine use, but also by the children's often chaotic home lives. The daily routine never varies, and unlike normal preschool and kindergarten classes, children are encouraged to develop strong attachments to teachers. This continuity and routine at school helps the children feel secure. Results are still inconclusive, but teachers are identifying instructional techniques to help these children with their drug-related developmental difficulties.

The efficacy of early intervention strategies for children with learning and emotional problems has been established (Dunst, Snyder, & Mankinen, 1986). The research findings previously described demonstrate that many cocaine-exposed children have real and persistent cognitive and social-emotional difficulties, which have serious implications for the unprepared school systems. Early intervention programs that will address the unique needs of this high-risk population are strongly recommended. Recommended intervention should include effective strategies for healthy development of these vulnerable children, as well as parent education. Table 3 lists some of the behavioral, learning, and developmental indiators for early intervention services because of perinatal substance abuse.

Parent Education

One important aspect of early intervention for cocaine-exposed children is the parent education component. For early intervention to be effective for this high-risk population, the service delivery system must be family oriented, and provide services that promote and support the parent's capability to be a good parent. Because many substance-abusing families come from diverse

Table 3. Perinatal Substance Abuse Developmental Indicators for Early Intervention Services

Type of Development	Indicators
Motor and neurological	Tremulousness, increased startling Poor quality of visual following Fine motor dexterity difficulty Blanking out, bizarre eye movements
Affective and behavioral	Depressed affect, decreased laughter Irritable, explosive, and impulsive behaviors Inability to self-regulate Marked difficulty with transition
Social/attachment	Decreased/absent stranger and separation anxiety Aggressiveness with peers Decreased response to verbal praise Decreased use of adults for solace
Language	Delayed acquisition of words Fewer spontaneous vocalizations from early infancy Difficulty in "word finding" at preschool level Decreased use of acquired words or gestures to communicate wants and needs
Problem solving and attention strategies	Poor on-task attention Increased distractibility to extraneous sounds and movements Inability to accommodate in problem solving situations Impulsive responses before "reflecting"

backgrounds, services should strive to meet the cultural and language needs of the families. Parent education should begin early enough so that parents can learn appropriate and effective caregiving.

Early intervention and treatment programs should strive not only to help the mothers deal with their addictions, but to teach them the parenting skills necessary for proper infant stimulation and subsequent development. Parents need to understand how easily the cocaine-exposed infant can become overstimulated. Parents need to be educated about fetal and infant development and the special needs of drug-exposed infants, as well as be given basic information about child nutrition and safety. Counseling may be necessary for crises and management of daily problems for parents and extended family.

Professionals who work with families must be aware of the danger of stereotyping. History of drug use patterns by mothers have different implications for parenting capacity. Moreover, not all babies exposed to cocaine in utero will be affected by the effects of cocaine, nor will those who are affected be affected in the same way. Stereotypes can blind professionals to the unique characteristics that both infants and mothers bring to their relationships, despite the impact of cocaine. Parent education must recognize, respect, and support individual differences, while addressing the very real risks that these mothers and infants face.

Several risk factors related to parenting appear to be more prevalent and can mitigate or exacerbate the adverse effects of in utero cocaine exposure. First, safety is a key issue since the cocaine-abusing parent often is unable to assume this primary protective role. Children often are in danger, because their addicted parents do not function as protectors and advocates. Often these children live in disruptive, chaotic environments where drugs are used and sold. Drive-by shootings and violence are daily occurrences in their neighborhoods. Therefore, the first goal of intervention is to monitor the child's safety.

An additional concern for children exposed to cocaine in utero is their risk for abuse, neglect, and placement in foster care. Regan, Ehrlich, and Finnegan (1987) found that histories of violence and/or abuse experienced by drug-dependent women far exceed that reported by a drug-free comparison group. Their findings suggest that there is a relationship between the occurrence of violence/abuse during childhood and subsequent drug abuse, and that the presence of drug abuse disrupts a woman's parenting ability. In addition, 40% of the drug-dependent sample had at least one child in some type of foster placement, or with relatives. This high number contributes to the swelling number of foster care placements. Currently, drug use is blamed for the growing number of children in foster care. Infants and very young children are entering foster care at a disproportionately high rate. In California, foster care placement increased 28% from 1986 to 1988 (Christie, Newbergh, Ghent, & Frost, 1989). More importantly, the number of drug-exposed infants entering foster care is creating a new set of demands upon foster families and social workers. According to Weston, Ivins,

Zuckerman, Jones, and Lopez (1989), the foster care system is so strained that many of these infants remain in hospitals for lack of homes deemed adequate to meet their extensive medical needs.

In summary, many children of cocaine abusing parents are living in unstable, dysfunctional, and often dangerous environments, cared for inconsistently by parents impaired by chronic drug use. According to Regan et al. (1987):

The markedly high incidence of abuse and violence in the lives of pregnant drug dependent women places them at high risk for parenting. Since these women are the primary caretakers, this is a major problem for themselves and their children. (p. 318)

The challenge facing clinicians, early interventionists, and researchers is to develop maternal/infant substance-abuse and health treatment programs that emphasize the impact of parenting on their children. Providers need to focus on more than the medical needs of the children and address the social and emotional needs of both infant and mother as well. Only through parent education and intervention, provided in a supportive, nonthreatening environment, will these mothers gain the skills necessary to foster healthy child development and realize that recovery is possible.

Impact on Professionals

Cocaine is taking an increasing toll on health care services, early intervention programs, foster care agencies, and other helping professions that deal with maternal/infant substance abuse. A whole new set of complex problems has been created for these professionals, coupled with a lack of resources and funds to deal with these youngest victims of the crack/cocaine epidemic. The prevalence of cocaine-exposed children has changed the very nature of many human services jobs, with interventions further complicated by issues of parenting ability, resources in the home, and basic safety. Follow-up is difficult, since substance-abusing parents are unstable, move frequently, lack telephones, fail to keep appointments, and drop out of sight when using illicit drugs. Protective service referrals and foster care placements become routine interventions. Early intervention specialists, social workers, Neonatal Intensive Care Unit (NICU) staff, and foster care agencies cope with heavy caseloads, spend a disproportionate amount of time searching for and contacting parents, and struggle to establish some sort of working alliance with them. According to Weston et al. (1989), many of these practitioners perceive the increased concentration of cocaine-exposed children as bringing higher stress to the effectiveness of their work, decreasing job satisfaction, and requiring new coping strategies.

Whatever the difficulties faced by professionals who treat cocaine- and other drug-exposed children and their families, few professionals have adequate preparation or resources to handle such a large proportion of high-risk cases. Educators fear that these children, including the estimated 375,000 drug-exposed children born annually (Miller, 1989), will overwhelm unprepared school systems. With the current trend toward a more academic kindergarten, these cocaine-exposed children may lag behind their normal peers. Eventually, these children will require special education. Special education is already underfunded and overloaded, and if the number of special education students swells because of the wave of these needy children, school districts most likely will face a severe financial crunch. This new wave of children placed in special education will only exacerbate the current shortage of special education teachers. Already, some school districts are experiencing the drug epidemic in the dramatic rise of special education referrals by hospitals, doctors, and county social workers. To accommodate these drug-exposed children, some school districts have added new, special education preschool classes (Christie et al., 1989).

More special training, administrative support, and in-services are required for educators to deal with the problems of drug-exposed children. This special training should encompass interagency and interdisciplinary training programs, including Child Protective Services, social services, corrections, drug and alcohol treatment, health care, mental health, and early intervention service providers to address the difficulties and training needed by these professionals. Service delivery programs must allow for ongoing supervision, consultation, and peer support so that problems, feelings, and particularly troublesome treatment issues can be shared. Staff support methods, including monitoring caseloads, respecting feelings of ineffectiveness, and staff education are essentials to prevent burnout and turnover. Foster care families also need support. By providing mental health services, respite care, training, financial incentives, and other support services for foster families, long-term placements and greater stability for these children may be ensured.

As America's cocaine problem worsens, professionals must prepare to deal with a steady stream of cocaine-exposed children. With the lack of resources and funds, the search for solutions will call for more creative and collaborative efforts. It is critical, then, that the recognition and ongoing discussion of the special difficulties faced by professionals who treat cocaine-exposed children and their families is continuous for the delivery of quality care.

The Challenge to Education

Public Law 99–457 establishes a program to provide early intervention services to infants and toddlers (birth through age 5) who are handicapped or developmentally delayed, and their families. To be eligible for services, the infant or toddler must be experiencing a developmental delay in one or more areas, or have a mental or physical condition with a high probability of resultant developmental delay. It appears, almost without doubt, that special education and those trained in early childhood education, mental health, and social services will be serving cocaine-exposed children, since this population meets the criteria outlined in P.L. 99–457.

Those with interest in special education and child development are beginning to realize the far-reaching effects that prenatal cocaine exposure has on children. Research in this area is urgently needed and should become a priority area for educational and developmental specialists. A plethora of questions pertaining to the impact of maternal cocaine use during pregnancy, long-term effects of in utero cocaine exposure on infant and child development, and its subsequent educational implications are ripe for study. The following discussion identifies areas of further research and the challenges presented to special educators, developmentalists, and others concerned with early childhood development.

A theoretical framework for the development of effective identification, prevention, and early intervention approaches to prenatal drug exposure needs to be developed. A conceptual framework based on a "risk model," rather than a "deficit model," needs to be addressed to assist clinical and research efforts. A deficit model for cocaine-exposed children and their families assumes that the difficulty of the child is attributed to the single cause of drug exposure; and the complexities of the impact of drugs on parents and children are deemed beyond understanding and preventive interventions — beyond professional help. With this assumption, a deficit model can be used to rationalize not providing services to cocaine-exposed children and their mothers (Weston et al., 1989).

On the other hand, a risk model recognizes that fetal exposure to cocaine compromises or jeopardizes developmental processes, but that environmental factors can contribute to positive developmental outcomes. Studies of vulnerable children have repeatedly indicated that developmental outcomes are the product of both heredity and environment, and that a dynamic, transactional model is needed (Sameroff & Chandler, 1975; Werner & Smith, 1982).

In addition, the need for a theoretical framework in which to conduct research is necessary to inform policy and practice. The testing of theories linking parental cocaine use to children's problems is necessary to identify what types of interventions are necessary. For example, developmental consequences for children may be related to the cocaine-abusing parents' family of origin, to the degree, amount, and type of drugs mothers ingested during pregnancy, or to the parenting responses to the child after birth. Findings from research designs developed to test theories from each of these perspectives can result in recommendations for service delivery model development and interventions that are likely to have a positive impact.

Furthermore, follow-up studies must look at intra-individual differences, rather than just intergroup differences, and realize that prenatal cocaine exposure is only one of many factors that contribute to risk. Factors such as the characteristics of the infant, the caretaking environment, abstinence effects, and so on, may cloud the picture and, therefore, should be considered in outcome studies. In addition, studies are needed to document motor development of cocaine-exposed infants later on in the first year of life. Follow-up of these infants through preschool and early school years will help identify any behavior or learning disorder that may be associated with prenatal cocaine exposure.

Research on the impact of either foster care or a drug-exposed environment, and the effect on the development of these infants, is needed. Research is difficult to do because of the problems of long-term follow-up and multiple confounding factors for this high-risk population. Studies of this type could yield valuable information for the more precise identification of populations at risk and the design of preventative treatment and intervention. In addition, studies of the parent-child interactions and the effectiveness of parent education for drug-abusing parents, including outcomes for the parent as well as the child, are needed.

With the epidemic of cocaine exploding onto the American landscape, drug abuse or drug addiction problems no longer affect only the individual, but have a devastating impact on infants, children, and families. Research, practice, and policy development relating to cocaine-exposed children and their families must reflect the support for optimal development for this heterogeneous population of children and families and must address their complex needs. This means that we need to place children and their parents as a priority, to integrate the information from multiple disciplines into a larger field of endeavor and share this information with others. A child's development relies on the coordination and collaboration of social, educational, and medical strategies which will ensure the healthy and orderly development of that child. The challenge for researchers and practitioners becomes one of learning how better to assist cocaine-exposed children and their families in identifying services that will prevent and remediate this social tragedy.

References

American Academy of Pediatrics. (1988). Cocaine emergency. *American Academy of Pediatric News, 14,* 3.

Burns, K., Melamed, J., Burns, W., Chasnoff, I., & Hatcher, R. (1986). Chemical dependency and depression in pregnancy. *Journal of Clinical Psychology, 41,* 851–854.

Burns, W. J. (1986). Psychopathology of mother-infant interaction. In I. J. Chasnoff (Ed.), *Drug use in pregnancy: Mother and child* (pp. 106-116). Norwell, England: Kluwer Academic Publishers.

Chasnoff, I. J. (Ed.). (1988). *Drugs, alcohol, pregnancy, and parenting.* London: Kluwer Academic Publishers.

Chasnoff, I. J. (1988, October). National Hospital Incidence Survey Perinatal Addiction Research and Education. *Update* (NAPARE Newsletter).

Chasnoff, I. J., Burns, K. A., & Burns, W. J. (1987). Cocaine use in pregnancy: Perinatal morbidity and mortality. *Neurotoxicology and Teratology, 9,* 291–293.

Chasnoff, I. J., Burns, W. J., Schnoll, S. H., & Burns, K. A. (1985). Cocaine use in pregnancy. *The New England Journal of Medicine, 313,* 666–669.

Chasnoff, I. J., & Griffith, D. R. (1989). Cocaine: Clinical studies of pregnancy and the newborn. *Annals of New York Academy of Sciences, 562,* 260–266.

Christie, A., Newbergh, C., Ghent, J., & Frost, J. (1989, May 25). Children in crisis. *The Oakland Tribune,* pp. 2–19.

Dunst, C. J., Snyder, S., & Mankinen, M. (1986). Efficacy of early intervention. In M. Wang, H. Walberg, & M. Reynolds (Eds.), *Handbook of special education: Research and practice* (Vol. 1–3). Oxford, England: Pergamon Press.

Finnegan, L. (1976). Clinical effects of pharmacologic agents on pregnancy, the fetus, and the neonate. *Annals of New York Academy of Science, 281,* 74.

Griffith, D. R. (1988). The effects of perinatal cocaine exposure on infant neurobehavior and early maternal-infant interactions. In I. J. Chasnoff (Ed.), *Drugs, alcohol, pregnancy and parenting* (pp. 105-114). London: Kluwer Academic Publishers.

Howard, J., Beckwith, L., Rodning, C., & Kropenske. V. (1989). The development of young children of substance-abusing parents: Insights from seven years of investigation and research. *Zero to Three, 9,* 8-12.

Kantrowitz, B., Wingert, P., De La Pena, N., Gordon, J., & Padgett, T. (1990, February 12). The crack children. *Newsweek,* pp. 62-63.

Kronstadt, D. (1989). *Pregnancy and cocaine addiction: An overview of impact and treatment.* Drug Free Pregnancy Project Far West Laboratory for Educational Research and Development, San Francisco, CA.

Miller, G. (1989). Addicted infants and their mothers. *Zero to Three, 9,* 20-23.

Osofsky, J. (1976). Neonatal characteristics and mother-infant interaction in two observational situations. *Child Development, 47,* 1138-1147.

Osofsky, J., & Danrger, B. (1974). Relationships between neonatal characteristics and mother-infant interaction. *Developmental Psychology, 10,* 124-130.

Pawl, J. (Ed.). (1989). Drug exposed babies [Special issue]. *Zero to Three, 9* (5).

Poulsen, M. K. (1989, December). *Risk factors in drug exposed infants and toddlers.* Paper presented at the meeting of the California Association of School Psychologists, Los Angeles, CA.

Regan, D. O., Ehrlich, S. M., & Finnegan, L. P. (1987). *Neurotoxicity and Teratology, 9,* 315-319.

Ryan, L., Ehrlich, S., & Finnegan, L. (1987). Cocaine abuse in pregnancy: Effects on the fetus and newborn. *Neurotoxicology and Teratology, 9, 295-299.*

Sameroff, A., & Chandler, M. J. (1975). Reproductive risk and the continuum of caretaking casualty. In F. D. Horowitz (Ed.), *Review of child development research* (Vol. 4, pp. 187-244). Chicago: University of Chicago Press.

Schneider, J. W. (1988). Motor assessment and parent education beyond the newborn period. In I J. Chasnoff (Ed.), *Drug use in pregnancy: Mother and child* (pp. 115-126). Norwell, England: Kluwer Academic Publishers.

Schneider, J. W., & Chasnoff, I. J. (1987). Cocaine abuse during pregnancy: Its effects on infant motor development — A clinical perspective. *Topics in Acute Care and Trauma Rehabilitation, 2,* 59-69.

Schneider, J. W., Griffith, D. R., & Chasnoff, I. J. (1989). Infants exposed to cocaine in-utero: Implications for developmental assessment and intervention. *Infants and Young Children, 2,* 25-36.

Smith, J. (1988). The dangers of prenatal cocaine use. *MCN, 13,* 174-179.

Werner, E., & Smith, R. (1982). *Vulnerable but invincible.* New York: McGraw-Hill.

Weston, D. R., Ivins, B., Zuckerman, B., Jones, C., & Lopez, R. (1989). Drug exposed babies: Research and clinical issues. *Zero to Three, 9,* 1-7.

Address correspondence to:
Sharon Lesar, Department of
Special Education, Graduate
School of Education, University of
California, Santa Barbara, CA 93106

Meeting the Needs of Children in Pennsylvania Who Are Exposed to Alcohol and Other Drugs

Anastasia Antoniadis, M.A., CCC/SLP
Eastern Instructional Support Center
King of Prussia, Pennsylvania

Deb Daulton, M.Ed.
Mid-State Instructional Support Center
Harrisburg, Pennsylvania

This article discusses how one state, Pennsylvania, has developed a mechanism for meeting the needs of children and families affected by alcohol and other drugs. Issues regarding women, dependency, and treatment and surveillance of children prenatally exposed to alcohol and other drugs are discussed. Act 212, Pennsylvania's Early Intervention Services System Act, is provided as an example of how this population of children and families can be better served through existing services and collaboration among state-level agencies.

Overview

Alcohol and other drug use, once considered an isolated problem, has now invaded the everyday lives of all people. The invasion comes not only from the impact of addiction on families, but also from the media's influence and coverage of this topic. Using the example of addiction to illegal drugs, one must approach the issue as an interplay of social, psychological, and biological factors influenced by financial, international, and political considerations (Turner, 1988). Consider the burden of cost to the health care system for managing the care of infants born exposed to cocaine (Coleman, 1991) in contrast to the profits gained by international drug trafficking endeavors. The median charge of hospitals to care for drug-exposed infants is $5,500 (per infant) compared to $1,400 for nonexposed infants (U.S. GAO Report, 1990). Profits

Infant-Toddler Intervention.
The Transdisciplinary Journal (Vol. 2, No. 1, pp. 53–62)
© 1992, Singular Publishing Group, Inc.

gained from the sale of illegal drugs, which frequently are reported in the billions, could pay for the care of these infants and the treatment programs required to assist their mothers in recovery from addiction. The economic impact of drug trafficking has been such that in 1988, two drug dealers were named on *Forbes'* list of the one hundred wealthiest individuals in the world. The economics of third-world countries are often dependent on the local drug trade. Thus, it comes as no surprise that there is heightened interest in the war on drugs by chief executive officers, politicians, and world leaders. The current mood in the United States has little tolerance for substance abuse, and it is influenced by an administration which advocates legal intervention as a means to end the "war on drugs."

Within this political and economic climate, however, the needs of the individual and family with addiction to alcohol and other drugs must not be lost. Central to the war on drugs are real people from all walks of life who share in the addiction-dependency experience. The real people we are talking about represent nearly half of the United States' population. It is estimated that over 102 million persons report current use of alcohol, over 10 million report current use of marijuana and hashish, and over 2 million report current use of cocaine or crack (NIDA, 1990).

Women, Babies, and Substance Abuse

Of growing concern is the use of alcohol and other drugs (AOD) among women, particularly women of childbearing age. An estimated 11% of pregnant women use AOD in this country (Miller, 1989). Although attention to the unique issues of women, addiction, and dependency is not new, only recently have these issues gained momen-

tum. Hagan (1987) found sexual assault, physical abuse, intergenerational addiction, and lack of family cohesion to be related significantly to addiction when comparing populations of drug-addicted and nonaddicted women from similar socioeconomic backgrounds. In traditional drug and alcohol treatment approaches, addicted women were being treated within a framework of a male model, that is, a model that was based on men's experiences with alcoholism. Neither women's life experiences or the influence of female physiology on addiction was taken into account. Speculation can be raised here as to whether the existence of male treatment models were due to economically driven discriminatory practices. For example, when the establishment of treatment programs for alcoholics began to multiply in the 1950s, they were designed for men because a man's decreased work productivity due to alcohol addiction was believed to have a greater impact on private industry and the economy at large than that of a woman's addiction problem. This viewpoint grew during an era when the number of women in the work force was significantly lower than what it is today. Therefore, treatment programs were designed to assist those individuals (i.e., men) who had more to contribute overall to the nation's economy.

Traditional treatment approaches that included women typically excluded those who were pregnant or who had young children (NCADD Policy Statement, 1990). Treatment centers lacked the appropriate staff to address the health care concerns of a pregnant addict. The staff's role was narrowly defined and did not consider the woman's role as a mother in the course of recovery. They also did not take into account cultural and ethnic factors that influence patterns of addiction unique to women. For example, drug preferences among women vary among Mexican-

Americans, Puerto Rican-Americans, and Cuban-Americans (Arkin & Funkhouser, 1990). Also, attitudes regarding drinking, drug addiction, gender roles, and the influence of religious practices on treatment are known to differ among Latino groups. As a result of these limitations to treatment, the needs of addicted women with or without children were not being met. Traditional approaches are being replaced slowly with new models. The creation of residential treatment programs as well as expanded outpatient services that treat both mother and child, and provide comprehensive services such as primary health care, adult literacy, vocational training, and parenting skills, has been fostered by state and federal grants. In 1985, 5% of federal dollars to states were set aside for the establishment of additional drug and alcohol treatment centers for women. In 1989, this figure increased to 10%. These changes were long overdue and much needed. To date, 24 programs, residential and nonresidential, that serve 152 women and 220 children have been implemented throughout Pennsylvania. While these numbers may be above the national average, there are waiting lists for the majority of inpatient centers statewide.

Of equal concern regarding the rise in AOD use in women of childbearing age is the rise of drug- and alcohol-related births. It is interesting to note that this concern has focused its efforts on the relationship of crack-cocaine, fetal development, and child outcome rather than alcohol use during pregnancy, which is far more insidious and difficult to document. From numerous reports found in professional literature, it is now well established that babies born to women who are frequent users of crack-cocaine are more likely to experience fetal strokes, small brain growth, low birthweight, and premature birth than babies born to non-using women (Chasnoff, 1989; Frank, 1990; Hadeed & Siegal, 1989; Keith et al.,

1989; Mitchell, et al., 1988). The fate of these infants once they enter school has yet to be understood fully. The first generation of children born since the crack epidemic began in 1985 are now entering public school. Based on limited research studies, it has been suggested that these children experience developmental delays through infancy and the preschool years (Griffith, 1990). Once in school, specific problem areas such as fine and gross motor clumsiness, delayed and exaggerated social-emotional reactions, and attentional difficulties have been identified (Bresnahan, Brooks, & Zuckerman, 1991; Howard, Beckwith, Rodning, & Kropenske, 1989).

Surveillance Issues in Pennsylvania

Accurately determining the incidence of drug-and alcohol-related births has been somewhat problematic. This is due, in part, to selective or biased reporting methods (Chasnoff, Landress, & Barrett, 1990). Another problem lies in the uniformity of reporting such births. Questions regarding drug- and alcohol-related births on revised birth certificates, for example, do not always yield accurate information. There may be underreporting due to lack of reliable information from maternal sources or from a hospital's records. Likewise, information from drug testing may be unreliable. In an article by O'Keefe (1987), mass drug screening identifies too many false positives, hence people are inappropriately being labeled as drug users. Staff responsible for completing birth certificate information may not be trained adequately to assess drug and alcohol use during pregnancy. Many hospitals do not have policies that regulate how to account for the number of drug- and alcohol-related births. Other hospitals do so using loosely defined criteria. Such was the case in 1990 when the Pennsylvania State

Health Data Center attempted to document incidence rates of drug- and alcohol-related births across the state (Pennsylvania Department of Health, 1991). Only 67% of all hospitals statewide were able to respond to survey questions regarding drug-related births. To further illustrate difficulties with surveillance, consider alcohol-related births resulting in fetal alcohol syndrome (FAS). FAS is considered the leading cause of preventable mental retardation in the United States and has an incidence rate of 1 in 750 to 1,000 live births. Its detection can be established more readily than other drug-related birth conditions due to the "recognized pattern of major and minor malformation, growth deficiency, and developmental disability caused by heavy alcohol exposure to utero" (Streissguth, 1986, p. 3). In spite of this, FAS is still considered an underreported condition, particularly during the neonatal period, because of lack of training in making the diagnosis (Little, Snell, Rosenfeld, Gilstrap, & Gant, 1990). For the year 1989, only 22 FAS cases were documented (from birth certificate information) in Pennsylvania while 224 FAS cases would have been expected based on the number of live births reported for the same year.[1] This discrepancy may be explained by the fact that, except for extreme cases, FAS characteristics may not be noticed at the time a birth certificate is filed for a particular infant, or diagnosis may not be possible at the time of hospital discharge.

Retrospective studies are utilized to document the number of alcohol- and drug-related births within a given time period. The need for careful interpretation of such data, however, must be respected. For example, cocaine use was found to occur in 16.3% of women delivering babies in selected Philadelphia hospitals by inspecting the hospital charts of all births in eight city hospitals during an 8-week period (Philadelphia Health Department, 1989). However, not all women and live babies born during this period were subject to an identical protocol for documenting the presence of alcohol or other drugs at the time of labor and delivery. Prevalence of other drug-related births in the United States, such as heroin, marijuana, and prescription drugs are reported to range from .4 to 27%. The current number of drug-related births overall (not including alcohol or tobacco use) has been estimated at 1 to 2% of all live births, or 40,000 to 75,000 per year (Cook, Petersen, & Moore, 1990). Caution must be exercised when using these figures because they may not accurately represent the total population of live births in the United States.

Recently, there have been a number of states that have passed legislation that mandates reporting of babies who screen positively for AOD. Mandated reporting is another example of how surveillance of AOD-related births can be maintained. There are a number of legal cases pending that challenge such legislation. A major argument presented by women's advocates is that such reporting constitutes a violation of the mother's civil rights. Another argument is that criminalization does not adequately deal with the real issues of a woman's addiction. That addiction is a health issue, not a legal issue, is an argument presented by those working in the mental health and health care fields. Paradoxically, child advocates do not necessarily view mandated reporting in the same way. One counterpoint presented by child advocates is that this type of reporting ensures a child's safety and welfare.

Caregiver Use and Effect on Child Outcome

The young child's environmental exposure to alcohol and other drugs, via family or care-

---

[1] In 1989, there were 168,108 resident live births recorded in Pennsylvania.

giver use, is an issue that, to date, has received little attention. A recent study conducted by the Philadelphia Department of Human Services concluded that children who were exposed to cocaine in their homes had more serious behavior problems than children whose exposure was limited to the prenatal period (Youngstrom, 1991). The potential for abuse in homes where there is active drug use is high. Among cases of child fatalities reported in Philadelphia, over half involved heavy parental use of cocaine (Hoerlin, 1989). It is apparent that not only is prenatal exposure to AOD detrimental to the child, but it also is detrimental when the exposure is chronic within the child's environment. Considering this from a transactional model of human development proposed by Horowitz (1985), as the child's environmental risk increases, so does the likelihood of poor developmental outcome. In other words, the prenatally exposed child already vulnerable at birth, has a decreased chance of a healthy developmental outcome if his or her environment is compromised by a caregiver who is abusing substances.

Consideration also must be given to the effect of caregiver use of AOD on child safety. Caregiver use of illegal drugs has resulted in accidental poisoning of young children (Dinnies, Darr, & Saulys, 1990). Recent attention has been given to the complications arising from passive inhalation of cocaine by infants and toddlers whose caregivers smoke crack (Bateman & Heagarty, 1989), exposure to infants during breast feeding (Chasnoff, Lewis, & Squires, 1985), and through accidental ingestion (Rivkin & Gilmore, 1989).

Pennsylvania's ACT 212

In December 1990, Act 212, The Early Intervention Services System Act, was signed into law in Pennsylvania. The following year, Pennsylvania created an entitlement program for all eligible young children and their families. All eligible children, birth through 2 years of age, would be entitled to early intervention services provided by the Pennsylvania Department of Public Welfare. Eligible children of this age group include children who are experiencing developmental delays or have a physical or mental condition that has a high probability of resulting in a developmental delay. Examples include Down syndrome and FAS. All eligible children, 3 years old to the "age of beginners" (the minimum age established by the school district board of directors for admission to the district's first grade) would be entitled to early intervention services provided by the Pennsylvania Department of Education. For 3- through 5-year-olds, eligibility includes children who have one of the physical or mental disabilities as defined in Part B of P.L. 102–119, the Individuals with Disabilities Education Act (formerly P.L. 94–142, the Education of the Handicapped Act), or who have a developmental delay as defined in the Pennsylvania Special Education Standards (Chapter 342).

Technically, many children who demonstrate neurological, social, and emotional or developmental delays as a result of the effects of alcohol or other drugs could have been served under Part B of the Education of the Handicapped Act if the delays were significant enough to meet state eligibility criteria. However, they typically were not served for a variety of reasons. Some of these reasons include failure to identify children affected by alcohol and other drugs, lack of advocacy, lack of sophisticated assessment devices in the social/emotional domain, and underfunding of the Act.

Pennsylvania's ACT 212, however, creates a different structure for the delivery of early intervention services. In addition to the eligible populations in Pennsylvania listed previously, Act 212 also mandates interagency collaboration to identify, screen, and track children birth through 5 years of age who are at risk. The purpose of this system is to identify those children who require specialized, more intensive services. The population groups eligible for these services are:

1. Children whose birthweight was less than 1,500 grams.
2. Children who experience a Neonatal Intensive Care Unit stay.
3. Children born to chemically dependent mothers.
4. Children who have experienced substantiated child abuse and neglect and are referred by the local children and youth agency.
5. Children with confirmed dangerous levels of lead poisoning as set by the Department of Health.

These criteria were selected in order to channel resources toward children who are known to be at increased risk of developing disabilities. The at-risk screening and tracking system creates a community-based service system for the delivery of identification, monitoring, and referral services. The necessity to identify and monitor these children and families who are not immediately eligible for services will provide a vehicle to consistently reevaluate progress and assist in obtaining status changes. Interagency coordination of data collection activities will strengthen the knowledge base regarding at-risk children as well as those eligible for services. The administrative agencies and community implementation open the door for new types of collaboration, advocacy, and models for program planning and implementation.

It is important to note the terminology used for eligibility for services under Pennsylvania law. Children with diagnosed conditions resulting in a high probability of developmental delay have presumptive eligibility for full entitlement services. This includes children with FAS, which is internationally recognized, and contributes to developmental delay (West, 1986). Children diagnosed with FAS are among those eligible from birth to 3 years of age. Children from 3 years old through the age of beginners are eligible under one of the categories of P.L. 102–119,[2] or as developmentally delayed. This discrepancy forces a comprehensive evaluation of the child with FAS at 3 years old to determine continued eligibility and bases this eligibility on the child's developmental needs rather than on a label of FAS.

Children eligible for tracking and monitoring include "children born to chemically dependent mothers." However, to become eligible for full entitlement they must be developmentally delayed or meet one of the P.L. 102–119 categories. The point worthy of note regarding the terminology is that Pennsylvania has not created a new category of "drug babies, crack children, or addicted infants." Categorization of this type would not be accurate as there is no homogeneous grouping or syndrome that readily identifies the effects of exposure to drugs in utero, nor is the methodology for specifying drug-specific behavioral or biologic outcome well developed. A category of "drug babies" is, therefore, inappropriate and provides no useful information based on the classification of children by such labels. In Pennsylvania, eligibility is based on developmental needs of children, assessed in terms of the child's and family's strenghths

---

[2] Categories include: mental retardation, hearing and visual impairments including blindness and deafness; speech or language impairments; serious emotional disturbances; orthopedic impairments; autism; traumatic brain injury; other health impairment; or specific learning disabilities.

and those things required to achieve optimal functioning.

Pennsylvania's Technical Assistance Program Serving Young Children and Families Affected by Alcohol and Other Drugs

In recognition of the increasing needs of children and families affected by alcohol and other drugs, and the professionals who serve them, Pennsylvania has begun to coordinate various federal programs at the state level. The Department of Education (Bureau of Special Education) and the Department of Public Welfare (the administrator of Part H of P.L. 102–119) have entered into a Memorandum of Understanding, which for the first time establishes a program devoted specifically to infants, toddlers, preschoolers, and their families affected by alcohol and other drugs, and women of child-bearing age at risk for abusing alcohol and other drugs. The initiative was developed to support two state consultants who will provide informational services and technical assistance to state departments, state organizations, and other service providers involved with women of child-bearing age, and families with young children affected by alcohol and other drugs.

Statewide Needs Assessment

The initial efforts of this initiative have been to assess the numbers and the needs of these populations in the communities in Pennsylvania. The needs assessment has been piloted in coordination with the Philadelphia Coordinated Health Care program with consultation from the U.S. Public Health Service, the Pennsylvania State Health Data Center, and the Temple University Institute on Disabilities. The provider survey and needs assessment have been piloted in 10 counties within the state which represent urban, suburban, and rural diversity. The questionnaire was designed to (1) assess providers' perceptions of the characteristics and needs of families and young children who are affected by alcohol and other drugs, (2) determine current referral patterns unique within communities, and (3) make recommendations about needed policies and programs. A preliminary analysis of the data suggests strong patterns of intergenerational drug abuse as well as physical and sexual abuse within this population of children and caregivers. Although drug abuse crosses all socioeconomic lines, the majority of providers are identifying families that are chronically affected by alcohol and other drugs as those in poverty, headed by a single unemployed, undereducated woman. Children are described by providers as exhibiting a range of characteristics. Speech and language and social-emotional delays are the most frequently reported characteristics.

An initial look at current referral patterns suggests that agencies whose primary clientele are children typically do not refer their families (whom they suspect have an addiction problem) to drug and alcohol treatment centers. Of those providers who do make referrals, several barriers faced by families to receive drug and alcohol treatment include waiting lists and client denial of their addiction problem. Likewise, drug and alcohol treatment centers typically do not refer clients with children to early intervention programs. In face-to-face interviews with the staff of these centers, one problem that has been identified is that they have not received sufficient awareness training regarding Pennsylvania Act 212 and how early intervention services may be accessed by children and families while in drug and alcohol treatment. Child welfare agencies (e.g., children and youth protective services, foster care services) appear to be most successful in making and receiving referrals to and from a wide range of providers outside of their own agency. While the results of the needs assessment are not fully analyzed, one might speculate that the reason for the successful referral patterns of child welfare agencies is due to their historical access of a variety of providers outside of their own, such as law enforcement, the courts, hospitals, schools, shelters, and drug and alcohol treatment centers. Other information from the needs assessment will be utilized to draft a report regarding service needs, program recommendations, and implementation strategies with their fiscal implications for state agencies and programs.[3]

Family Focused Early Intervention System (FFEIS)

This program, drawing from Act 212 funds, is newly created in Pennsylvania. The FFEIS is designed to train families and providers of early childhood and early intervention services throughout the state at the community level. The identification of training needs pivots around local interagency coordinating councils, whose role will be to determine the needs, level of training, and composition of their community agency members. State consultants serving within Pennsylvania's Instructional Support System, including alcohol and other drug technical assistance programs, are responsible for working with local communities, development of training modules, and implementation of training workshops to agency personnel, intermediate units, school districts, families, nursery schools, and preschools. Because families will receive training side by side with professionals, the modules will be broad in focus, enabling trainers to meet the needs of a diverse target audience. Content areas for alcohol and other drug modules will include fetal alcohol syndrome and fetal alcohol effects, illicit and prescription drug use and their impact on child development, inclusion and sensitivity issues regarding children affected by alcohol and other drugs in the classroom, and family cultural aspects of addiction and dependency. When fully implemented, this training initiative will have a major impact on services to young children and their families and to professionals working in the early childhood and early intervention fields.

Summary

Alcohol and other drug use affect young children and families in unique and insidious ways. To meet the special needs of this population, Pennsylvania has chosen to utilize existing funds within early intervention to create technical assistance and training to a diverse audience of state agencies and local service providers. This was made possible by the collaboration of state Departments of Education and Welfare and their commitment to serving young children and families affected by alcohol and other drugs. Collaboration among a wider variety of state and local systems will be the next challenge as we face the long and arduous road to recovery and wellness for Pennsylvania's most vulnerable citizens.

Acknowledgments

The authors wish to thank the Pennsylvania Department of Education (Bureau of Special Education and Bureau of Basic Education Support Services) and Public Welfare (Office of Mental Retardation) for their

---

[3] A peer review of this document is being planned for later this year.

support of the program described in this article. The authors also wish to recognize Ms. Penny Ettinger of Philadelphia Coordinated Health Care, Dr. Alden Small of the Pennsylvania State Health Data Center, Dr. James Conroy of Temple University, and James Binkley of the Mid-State Instructional Support Center who have provided technical assistance to this program. Additional acknowledgments are extended to the Instructional Support System of Pennsylvania and the following Intermediate Units: IU #13 (Lancaster–Lebanon), IU #16 (Central Susquehanna), and IU #23 (Montgomery County).

References

Arkin, E. B., & Funkhouser, J. E. (Eds.). (1990). Communicating about alcohol and other drugs: Strategies for reaching populations at risk. *OSAP Prevention Monograph-5*. DHHS Publication No. (ADM)90-1665, pp. 175–177.

Bateman, D. A., & Heagarty, M. C. (1989). Passive freebase cocaine ('Crack') inhalation by infants and toddlers. *American Journal of Diseases in Children, 143*, 25–27.

Bresnahan, K., Brooks, C., & Zuckerman, B. (1991). Prenatal cocaine use: Impact on infants and mothers. *Pediatric Nursing, 17*, 123–129.

Chasnoff, I. J. (1989). Cocaine, pregnancy, and the neonate. *Women and Health, 15*, 23–35.

Chasnoff, I. J., Landress, H. J., & Barrett, M. E. (1990). The prevalence of illicit-drug or alcohol use during pregnancy and discrepancies in mandatory reporting in Pinellas County, Florida. *The New England Journal of Medicine, 322*(17), 1202–1206.

Chasnoff, I. J., Lewis, D. E., & Squires, L. (1985). Cocaine intoxication in a breast-fed infant. *Pediatrics, 80*, 836–838.

Coleman, B. C. (1991). Study: Cost high for hospitalizing cocaine infants. *Philadelphia Inquirer*, October 14, p. A-2.

Cook, P., Petersen, R. C., & Moore, D. T. (1990). Alcohol, tobacco, and other drugs may harm the unborn. DHHS Publication No. (ADM) 90-1711.

Dinnies, J. D., Darr, C. D., & Saulys, A. J. (1990). Cocaine toxicity in toddlers. *American Journal of Diseases in Children, 144*, 743–744.

Frank, D. A. (1990, August). *Infants of substance abusing mothers: Demographics and medical profile.* Paper presented at the Babies and Cocaine Conference, Washington, DC.

Griffith, D. (1990, August). *The effects of perinatal drug exposure on child development: Implications for early intervention and education.* Paper presented at the Babies and Cocaine Conference, Washington, DC.

Hadeed, A., & Siegal, S. (1989). Maternal cocaine use during pregnancy: Effect on the newborn infant. *Pediatrics, 82*, 888–895.

Hagan, T. A. (1987). A retrospective search for the etiology of drug abuse: A background comparison of a drug-addicted population of women and a control group of non-addicted women. *NIDA Research Monograph Series of Health and Human Services.*

Hoerlin, B. Y. (1989). *Connecting: Challenges in health and human services in the Philadelphia region.* Philadelphia, PA: The Pew Charitable Trusts.

Horowitz, F. D. (1985). Making a model of development and its implications for working with young infants. *Zero to Three, 6*, 1–13.

Howard, J., Beckwith, L., Rodning, C., & Kropenske, V. (1989). The development of young children of substance-abusing parents: Insights from seven years of intervention research. *Zero to Three, 9*, 8–12.

Keith, L. G., MacGregor, S., Friedell, S., Rosner, M., Chasnoff, I. J., & Sciarra, J. J. (1989). Substance abuse in pregnant women: Recent experience at the Perinatal Center for Chemical Dependence of Northwestern Memorial Hospital. *Obstetrics and Gynecology, 73*, (5, Pt. I), 715–719.

Little, B. B., Snell, L. M., Rosenfeld, C. R., Gilstrap, L. C., & Gant, N. F. (1990). Failure to recognize Fetal Alcohol Syndrome in newborn infants. *American Journal of Diseases in Children, 144*, 1142–1146.

Miller, G. (1989). Addicted infants and their mothers. *Zero to Three, 9*, 20–23.

Mitchell, M., Sabbagha, R., Keith, L., MacGregor, S., Mota, J., & Minoque, J. (1988). Ultrasonic growth parameter in fetuses of mothers with primary addiction to cocaine. *American Journal of Obstetrics and Gynecology, 159,* 1104–1109.

National Council on Alcoholism and Drug Dependence. (1990). *Women, alcohol, other drugs and pregnancy.* Policy statement.

National Institute on Drug Abuse, (1990). *Population estimates of lifetime and current drug use.* DHHS Publication No. C-84-3.

O'Keefe, A. N. (1987). The case against drug testing. *Psychology Today, 21,* 34–38.

Pennsylvania Department of Health. (1991). Drug-related births also a problem in Pennsylvania. *Statistical News from the State Health Data Center, 14,* 7.

Philadelphia Health Department. (1989). *One thousand babies: Philadelphia, 1989.* Unpublished report.

Rivkin, M., & Gilmore, H. E. (1989). Generalized seizures in an infant due to environmentally acquired cocaine. *Pediatrics, 84,* 1100–1102.

Streissguth, A. P. (1986). The behavioral teratology of alcohol: Performance, behavioral, and intellectual deficits in prenatally exposed children. In J. West (Ed.), *Alcohol and brain development* (pp. 3–44). New York: Oxford University Press.

Turner, C. E. (1988). The cocaine epidemic and prevention of future drug epidemics. *Psychiatric Annals, 18*(9), 511–512.

United States General Accounting Office. (1990). Drug-exposed infants: A generation at risk. U.S. Government Printing Office, HRD-90-138.

West, J. (Ed.). (1986). *Alcohol and brain development.* New York: Oxford University Press.

Youngstrom, N. (1991). Drug exposure in home elicits worst behaviors. *APA Monitor, 22,* 23.

Address correspondence to:
A. Antoniadis
E-ISC
200 Anderson Road
King of Prussia, PA 19406

Language and Behavioral Concerns for Drug-Exposed Infants and Toddlers

Kenyatta O. Rivers, M.A.
University of Florida
Gainesville, Florida

Dona Lea Hedrick, Ph.D.
University of Central Florida
Orlando, Florida

This article presents information related to the language behaviors seen in children who had been prenatally exposed to cocaine. Eight speech-language pathologists provided descriptions on the language behaviors seen in these children according to four age groups. Related information, such as (1) the number of children prenatally exposed to cocaine being seen by speech-language pathologists (SLP) in three different settings, (2) the diagnostic tools and procedures used in diagnosing language deficits, and (3) the relationship of the caregivers who typically are custodians of children prenatally exposed to cocaine was gathered also. The most important finding was that children prenatally exposed to cocaine exhibit marked receptive and expressive language deficits. Receptive and expressive deficits were described as variable within and across age groups, but deficiencies sometimes become more subtle with each successive age group.

For some time there has been a considerable amount of research directed toward describing the behaviors of children exposed to substances via maternal use, particularly alcohol (Coles, Smith, & Falek, 1987; Gusella & Fried, 1984; Kaye, Elkind, & Tytun, 1989). However, research focusing on the children who have been prenatally exposed to cocaine has not been as abundant (Chasnoff, Lewis, Griffith, & Willey, 1989b; Frank et al., 1988; Griffith, 1988). For example, the behavioral characteristics of fetal alcohol syndrome will be discussed first because of the limited nature of the information on cocaine abuse. In addition, some behavioral characteristics may be in common.

Infant-Toddler Intervention.
The Transdisciplinary Journal (Vol. 2, No. 1, pp. 63–73)
© 1992, Singular Publishing Group, Inc.

The Effects of Prenatal Alcohol and Cocaine Exposure

Fetal Alcohol Syndrome (FAS)

Many researchers have reported on the behavioral characteristics of children maternally exposed to alcohol, which often is referred to as fetal alcohol syndrome (FAS) (Church & Gerkin, 1988; Fried & Watkinson, 1988). FAS often is defined as defects that are seen in children postnatally, such as central nervous system dysfunction, growth deficiencies, and mental alterations, which are the result of maternal alcoholism throughout the prenatal period (Thomas, 1985).

As infants, the manifestations of FAS are seen in children's decreased abilities to become accustomed to frequently occurring stimuli, less capable of becoming excited, and increased irritability (Church & Gerkin, 1988; Fried & Watkinson, 1988). Furthermore, weak sucking abilities and other feeding difficulties are other frequently mentioned characteristics of infants with FAS.

Children with FAS often show a decrease in their ability to realize that objects are relatively permanent and not destroyed if they are removed from one's visual field. In addition, they exhibit decreased memory and problem-solving skills, and they often exhibit a delay in the production of words (Fried & Watkinson, 1988).

Shaywitz, Caparulo, and Hodgson (1981) noted that children with FAS often have poor attention spans and display poor verbal abilities. With regard to speech and language abilities, the proper ordering of words in sentences (syntax) and the use of the correct meanings of words (semantics) are often in error. In addition, inappropriate use of language as a means of initiating and continuing social discourse is commonly seen.

Gusella and Fried (1984) stated that children exposed to alcohol in utero often exhibit central nervous system dysfunctions, growth deficiencies, and various facial anomalies and malformations. These authors further state that the most significant problem associated with prenatal alcohol exposure is mental retardation.

With regard to growth deficiencies, Sparks (1984) notes that growth deficiencies are a result of a diminished number of cells. Sparks states the following:

Growth deficiencies are most striking in brain and eye development than in linear growth and more pronounced in midfacial growth than in general skeletal growth. FAS children are born small for their gestational age with a head size that is reduced even in relation to their reduced length. Postnatally, these children continue to grow at a slow pace and tend to become underweight for their length. (p. 28)

Unlike the literature on FAS, the literature pertaining to in utero cocaine exposure and later outcomes on children has been relatively inconclusive with regard to potential outcomes. There are few consistent behaviors and characteristics that are typical of the majority of the children prenatally exposed to cocaine via maternal use.

Cocaine Exposure

Chasnoff et al. (1989b) and MacGregor et al. (1987) noted that infants exposed to cocaine tend to have decreased birthweights and head circumferences when compared to nonmaternally exposed infants. In addition, they are at risk for growth retardation.

Chasnoff et al. (1989b) state that infants exposed to cocaine often demonstrate deficiencies in their abilities to move adaptively through the various states of arousal in attending to and in actively engaging auditory and/or visual stimuli. Furthermore, they can be overloaded easily by environmental stimuli. As a result, they use various patterns of sleep and cry states to limit the amount of external stimuli that they will receive.

Fulroth, Phillips, and Durand (1989) noted that infants maternally exposed to cocaine often display hypertonia, hyperactive moro reflex, abnormal rapidity of respiration, loose stools, decreased sleep, excessive sucking, and nasal stuffiness. In addition, these infants are at risk for an abnormal rapidity of heart action. As a result, there is a high potential for cardiorespiratory abnormalities (Chasnoff, Hunt, Kletter, & Kaplan, 1989a; MacGregor et al., 1987). Fulroth et al. (1989) further noted that prenatal cocaine exposure often is associated with "growth retardation, microcephaly (abnormal smallness of the head; Thomas, 1985), and prematurity (p. 910)."

Howard (1989) noted that some children who are exposed prenatally to cocaine exhibit abnormal psychological behaviors. Howard suggested that the abnormal psychological behaviors that are seen in children prenatally exposed to cocaine are a result of cocaine's psychophysiological properties. In other words, neurophysiological changes of the brain stem may occur if it is continually exposed to cocaine (Howard, 1989). Therefore, behaviors such as chronic mood swings and irritability may be indicative of some neuronal impairments that were created via prenatal exposure to cocaine (Howard, 1989).

Howard (1989) noted that it is difficult for researchers to state precisely "how prenatal drug exposure and postnatal child-rearing environments interact and contribute to distortions in social-emotional development (p. 256)." However, Howard asserted that even though the precise interaction between cocaine and the environment is unknown, researchers should not diminish the implications of cocaine's role and impact on the neuropsychological systems of infants.

Research Questions

This pilot investigation was undertaken to address several questions related to the language behaviors associated with children maternally exposed to cocaine. The questions were as follows:

1. In what setting are speech-language pathologists more likely to see children who have been maternally exposed to cocaine?
2. How many of the children maternally exposed to cocaine were in the custodianship of a foster home care system [i.e., Health and Rehabilitative Services (HRS)], parents, relatives other than parents, or some other caregiver?
3. How many maternally exposed cocaine children are seen by speech-language pathologists for treatment, diagnosis, or treatment/diagnosis?
4. What are the language and cognitive behaviors exhibited by the cocaine-exposed children according to age group?
5. How do children who have been exposed prenatally to cocaine compare to the known consequences of alcohol on children?

Method of Data Collection

Eight speech-language pathologists (SLP) from Orlando, Florida, served as subjects for this study. The SLP held certificates of clinical competence (C.C.C.) from the American Speech-Language-Hearing Association (ASHA). These clinicians practiced in one of three settings. The settings and number of clinicians in each setting were as follows: private practice, 3; public schools, 4; and hospital, 1.

The clinicians who participated in this study provided treatment to and/or diagnosed children from the ages of birth to 12 years. The children in these caseloads exhibited various speech and language delays and disorders as a result of known and unknown etiological causes, including those who had been maternally exposed to cocaine.

The clinicians provided responses to nine questions on a survey form via interviews with the first author in their respective job settings. The survey form contained questions pertaining to the work settings and the number of children treated and/or diagnosed in each clinicians caseload. There also were questions that dealt with the number of children maternally exposed to cocaine in the clinicians' caseloads per week and per year and the types of services being rendered, such as treatment, diagnosis, or both.

The survey form included questions that inquired about the custodianship of the children prenatally exposed to cocaine and how the clinicians first became aware that their clients had been exposed to cocaine. Furthermore, there were questions pertaining to the assessment tools and procedures most frequently used to verify speech and language patterns, as well as the specific patterns and behaviors seen according to four age groups. The questionnaire that was used in this study is in the appendix.

Results of the Survey

Number of Children Seen Per Setting

As can be seen in Table 1, the number of children that data were presented on by the clinicians was 50. Seventy-two percent (N = 36) were seen in the public schools within a year for speech and language disorders and delays. In the private practice and hospital settings, 18% (N = 9) and 12% (N = 6) of the children were being diagnosed and/or treated, respectively, per year.

Who Has Custodianship?

Twenty-two of the children (44%) were reported to have been in the custody of HRS (i.e., foster homes). Eighteen (36%) of the children were reported to have been in the custody of other relatives, not the biological parents, and only 10 (20%) were with one or both parents.

Table 1. The work settings of speech-language pathologists and the total number of maternally cocaine-exposed children they see per week and per year

	N	Number of Children in Caseload per Week	Number of Cocaine Children Seen per Week	Number of Cocaine Children Seen per Year
Private	3*	85	2	9
School	4	42**	7**	36
Hospital	1	20	2	6

* Includes private practitioners and speech-language pathologists working in private agencies.
** These are approximate numbers. Two speech-language pathologists in this setting stated that the number of children in these categories varied from week to week.

How Clinicians Became Aware of Cocaine Exposure

The results of the survey indicated that the clinicians became aware that their clients had been exposed prenatally to cocaine via a combination of hospital reports, relatives other than biological parents, and other sources, primarily HRS. Clinicians seldom were made aware of the exposure via the biological parents, and none were made aware of the cocaine exposure via a family physician.

Frequently Used Diagnostic Tools

As can be seen in Table 2, the most frequent diagnostic tools used by the clinicians were the following: the *Sequenced Inventory of Communication Development — Revised* (SICD; Hedrick, Prather, & Tobin, 1984), the *Preschool Language Assessment Instrument* (PLAI; Blank, Rose, & Berlin, 1978), the *Expressive One-Word Picture Vocabulary Test* (EOWPVT; Gardner, 1979), the *Assessment of Children's Language Comprehension* (ACLC; Foster, Giddan, & Stark, 1973), and the *Test for Auditory Comprehension of Language — Revised* (TACL-R; Carrow-Woolfolk, 1985). In addition, all of the clinicians used language samples and informal observations of play to assist in their diagnosis of language delays and disorders.

The term "language delayed" often is used to refer to the language behaviors of children who are following a normal developmental pattern, but they are at a stage that is lower than one would expect given a child's chronological age. The term "language disordered" often is used to refer to the language behaviors of children who are

Table 2. Assessment tools and procedures used in diagnosing language deficits of maternally exposed cocaine children

Name	Number of Clinicians Using the Tool
Sequenced Inventory of Communication Development — Revised (SICD; Hedrick, Prather, & Tobin, 1984)	3
Preschool Language Assessment Instrument (PLAI; Blank, Rose, & Berlin, 1978)	3
Expressive One-Word Picture Vocabulary Test (EOWPVT; Gardner, 1979)	2
Goldman-Fristoe Test of Articulation (Goldman & Fristoe, 1972)	1
Receptive-Expressive Emergent Language Scale (REEL; Bzoch & League, 1971)	1
Preschool Language Scale (PLS; Zimmerman, Steiner, & Pond, 1979)	1
Assessment of Children's Language Comprehension (ACLC; Foster, Giddan, & Stark, 1973)	2
Illinois Test of Psycholinguistic Abilities (ITPA; Kirk, McCarthy, & Kirk, 1968)	1
Prutting Pragmatic Protocol (PPP; University of California, 1982)	1
Test of Problem Solving (TOPS; Zachman, Jorgensen, Huisingh, & Barrett, 1984)	1

(continued)

Table 2 (continued)

Name	Number of Clinicians Using the Tool
Test for Auditory Comprehension of Language — Revised (TACL—R; Carrow-Woolfolk, 1985)	2
Structured Photographic Expressive Language Test — II (SPELT-II; Werner & Kresheck, 1983)	1
Peabody Picture Vocabulary Test — Revised (PPVT—R; Dunn & Dunn, 1981)	1
Denver Developmental Screening Test (Frankenberg & Dodds, 1967)	1
Observation of Play	5
Language Sample	5

using language patterns that are atypical of the language patterns that one would expect a child to be using at any stage of the language development continuum.

Characteristic Behaviors By Age Levels

Birth to 2 Years

The following characteristics and behaviors are based on nine children. The most striking findings reported by the SLP with reference to children in this age group were the lack of oral language abilities and inappropriate use of gestures. Seventy-seven percent (N = 7) of the children were reported to have limited or no expressive language. Of the nine children reported on, two used consistent sound combinations to represent objects, but the sound combinations were very limited and often unintelligible.

All of the children used gestures. However, the clinicians noted that the gestures that were used were not always appropriate, and that the gestures seldom had any accompanying vocalizations. Social interactions were limited to denials with occasional requests.

With regard to cognition, it was reported that the children in this age group exhibited attention deficits, unusual behavior patterns (i.e., excessive crying, repetitious use of toys and objects with little variance), and decreased problem-solving skills. All of the children were described as not being able to maintain gains made in treatment sessions from one to the next if there were extended amounts of time between sessions.

It was noted that the children often showed low muscle tone and rapid mood swings. Furthermore, they were not consoled easily using normal techniques for comforting (i.e., holding, rocking) when they were crying.

2.1 to 4 Years

The following characteristics and behaviors are based on data that were provided on 25 children. Deficits were noted in the retrieval of words (i.e., verbs, names of people), in the naming of colors, and in counting using a numerical system. In addition, many of the children were noted as being unable to use concepts, such as hard and soft.

Syntactical skills, defined as the ordering of words in a sentence, tended to vary from one child to the next, but it was reported that approximately 50% of the children in this age group used sentences that were very disorganized (sequencing). In addition, sentence length typically varied between two and three words.

Pragmatic skills, which are defined by Rossetti (1991) as the ways in which one uses language as opposed to the ways in which language is designed, varied from mild to severe in severity, with poor eye contact and lack of turn taking being very common problems. Four of the eight clinicians reported that some of the children exhibited an increased amount of talkativeness and limited relatedness to others, whereas other children were described as being detached and superficial in relatedness.

Cognitively, the children varied from mild to severe in retardation. All of the children were characterized as being hyperactive and having decreased attention spans. Eighty-eight percent of the children were described as being very manipulative, and they often became absorbed with an activity. Therefore, clinicians reported that these children had problems with shifting from one task to another. Clinicians also noted that if changes in therapy were not made gradually, these children were likely to become overstimulated. As a result, cooperation and participation decreased.

4.1 to 6 Years

The characteristics provided in this age group are based on the behaviors exhibited by 14 children. These children's vocabularies were described as being very limited. They had difficulty with abstract concepts, multiple meaning words, and temporal/spatial concepts.

Sentences produced by these children were described as being simple, not complex (i.e., few dependent clauses). Furthermore, these children were described as having difficulties interacting appropriately with other children. However, they showed better eye contact and turn-taking skills in

comparison to those children in the 2- to 4-year age group.

Cognitively, these children were reported as having reduced attention spans, being very impulsive, and easily distracted. In addition, task shifting was often difficult.

The clinicians reported that such children are often classified in the school system as being learning disabled or emotionally handicapped. Therefore, they often are assigned to classroom environments that provide low levels of stimulation to keep overloading from occurring.

6.1 Years and Older

The characteristics provided in this section are based on the behaviors exhibited by two children. These children were reported as demonstrating word retrieval problems as seen in their inappropriate labeling of objects and people. In addition, their ordering of sentence elements were described as being disorganized. Therefore, when using their language skills in various contexts and situations, they often are described as being very difficult to understand or as being pragmatically inappropriate.

Short attention spans, problems with staying on task, and having low tolerance for changes made in their environments were descriptions used to refer to these children's cognitive abilities. Multiple articulation problems were noted. Moreover, the children in this group often were reported as showing poor interaction skills with other children.

Discussion

The most striking behaviors noted in this study were the marked delays in receptive and expressive language skills. Many of the deficits that were noted may prove to be significant when the possible influence of environmental factors is accounted for. Therefore, the behaviors that were reported may be indicative of a popula-tion of children who are at very high risk for primary central nervous system aberrations.

Children with FAS often are described as exhibiting behaviors that may be seen as typical of the majority of these children. In comparison to children with FAS, the children that were exposed prenatally to cocaine that were described in this study exhibited few behaviors that were characteristic of all of the children in the respective age groups. For example, 78% (N = 7) of the children in the birth to 2-year age group were described as not having any expressive language skills. However, 22% (N = 2) of the children in this group did produce various sound combinations, but the combinations were often limited and unintelligible. In another example, 88% (N = 22) of the children in the 2- to 4-year age group were described as having reduced sentence lengths (two to three words), but only 52% (N = 13) of the children were reported to have sentences that were disorganized (i.e., sequencing). Those children that were described in this study who were considered to have normal mental abilities and skills often were described as exhibiting subtle receptive and expressive language delays.

Structural malformations and aberrations (i.e., insufficient eye development, small head circumference) are often cited in the literature with regard to children with FAS. However, there were no prevailing physical differences that were reported consistently. Therefore, children prenatally exposed to cocaine seem to exhibit variations in language abilities, mental skills, and physical profiles.

Another finding of importance was that the SLP often stated that there appear to be problems with the transmittance of records and information from one professional to another and from one agency to another. It often was mentioned that reports citing that a given child was the product of a cocaine pregnancy are not always made available or not kept. As a result, other professionals and agencies are not receiving information that is pertinent to the proper treatment of children maternally exposed to cocaine. Therefore, SLP should attempt to acquire in-depth case history data.

In the future, there needs to be more detailed scientific research that focuses on the frequency of language and cognitive deficits associated with in utero cocaine exposure. In addition, the specific deficits that are seen need to be described.

Acknowledgments

The authors would like to thank Dr. Kenneth R. Bzoch for his comments and suggestions on this article.

References

Blank, M., Rose, S., & Berlin, L. (1978). *Preschool Language Assessment Instrument.* New York: Grune & Stratton.

Bzoch, K. R., & League, R. (1971). *Receptive Expressive Emergent Language Scale.* Austin, TX: Pro-Ed.

Carrow-Woolfolk, E. (1985). *Test of Auditory Comprehension of Language — Revised.* Boston, MA: DLM Teaching Resources.

Chasnoff, I. J., Hunt, C. E., Kletter, R., & Kaplan, D. (1989a). Prenatal exposure is associated with respiratory pattern abnormalities. *American Journal of Diseases of Children, 143* (5), 583–587.

Chasnoff, I. J., Lewis, D. E., Griffith, D. R., & Willey, S. (1989b). Cocaine and pregnancy: Clinical and toxicological implications for the neonate. *Clinical Chemistry, 35* (7), 1276–1278.

Church, M. W., & Gerkin, K. P. (1988). Hearing disorders in children with fetal alcohol syndrome: Findings from case reports. *Pediatrics, 82* (2), 147–154.

Coles, C. D., Smith, I. E., & Falek, A. (1987). Prenatal alcohol exposure and infant behavior: Immediate effects and implications for later development. *Advances in Alcohol and Substance Abuse, 6* (4), 87–104.

Dunn, L. M., & Dunn, L. M. (1981). *Peabody Picture Vocabulary Test — Revised.* Minneapolis, MN: American Guidance Service.

Foster, R., Giddan, J., & Stark, J. (1973). *Assessment of children's language comprehension.* Palo Alto, CA: Consulting Psychologists Press.

Frank, D. A., Zuckerman, B. S., Amaro, H., Aboague, K., Bauchner, H., Cabral, H., Fried, L., Hingson, R., Kayne, H., Levenson, S. M., Parker, S., Reece, H., & Vinci, R. (1988). Cocaine use during pregnancy: Prevalence and correlates. *Pediatrics, 82* (6), 888–895.

Frankenberg, W. K., & Dodds, J. B. (1967). *The Denver Developmental Screening Test.* Denver: University of Colorado Medical Center.

Fried, P. A., & Watkinson, B. (1988). 12- and 24-month neurobehavioral follow-up of children prenatally exposed to marihuana, cigarettes, and alcohol. *Neurotoxicology and Teratology, 10,* 305–313.

Fulroth, R., Phillips, B., & Durand, D. J. (1989). Perinatal outcome of infants exposed to cocaine and/or heroin in utero. *American Journal of Diseases in Childhood, 143,* 905–910.

Gardner, M. F. (1979). *Expressive One-Word Picture Vocabulary Test.* Novato, CA: Academic Therapy Publications.

Goldman, R., & Fristoe, M. (1972). *Goldman-Fristoe Test of Articulation.* Circle Pines, MN: American Guidance Service, Inc.

Griffith, D. R. (1988). The effect of perinatal exposure to cocaine on infant neurobehavior and early maternal-infant interaction. In I. J. Chasnoff (Ed.), *Drugs, alcohol, pregnancy and parenting.* Lancaster, UK: Kluwer Academic Publishers.

Gusella, J. L., & Fried, P. A. (1984). Effects of maternal social drinking and smoking on offspring at 13 months. *Neurobiological Toxicology and Teratology, 6,* 13–17.

Hedrick, D. L., Prather, E. M., & Tobin, A. R. (1984). *Sequenced Inventory of Communication Development — Revised.* Seattle, WA: University of Washington Press.

Howard, J. (1989). Cocaine and its effects on the newborn. *Developmental Medicine and Child Neurology, 31,* 255–257.

Kaye, K., Elkind, G., & Tytun, A. (1989). Birth outcomes for infants of drug abusing mothers. *New York State Journal of Medicine, 89,* 256–261.

MacGregor, S. N., Keith, L. G., Chasnoff, I. J., Rosner, M. A., Chisum, G. M., Shaw, P., & Minogue, J. P. (1987). Cocaine use during pregnancy: Adverse perinatal outcome. *American Journal of Obstetrics and Gynecology, 157* (3), 686–690.

McCarthy, K. S., & Kirk, W. (1968). *Illinois Test of Psycholinguistic Abilities.* Los Angeles, CA: Western Psychological Services.

Rossetti, L. M. (1991). Infant-toddler intervention assessment: A clinical perspective. *Infant-Toddler Intervention. 1* (1), 11–25.

Shaywitz, S. E., Caparulo, B. K., & Hodgson, E. S. (1981). Developmental language disability as a consequence of prenatal exposure to ethanol. *Pediatrics, 68* (6), 850–855.

Sparks, S. N. (1984). Speech and language in fetal alcohol syndrome. *American Speech, Language, and Hearing Association, 26* (2), 27–31.

Thomas, C. L. (Ed.). (1985). *Taber's cyclopedic medical dictionary* (16th Ed.). Philadelphia: F. A. Davis Company.

University of California. (1982). *Prutting pragmatic protocol.* Berkeley, CA: University of California.

Werner, E. O., & Kresheck, J. D. (1983). *Structured Photographic Expressive Language Test — II.* Sandwich IL: Janelle Publications, Inc.

Zachman, L., Jargensen, C., Hinusingh, R., & Barrett, M. (1984). *Test of problem solving.* Moline, IL: Lingui Systems.

Zimmerman, I. L., Steiner, V. G., & Pond, R. E. (1979). *Preschool Language Scales.* New York: Psychological Corporation.

Address correspondence to:
Mr. Kenyatta O. Rivers, M.A.,
Department of Communication
Processes and Disorders,
University of Florida, Dauer Hall,
Gainesville, FL 32611.

Appendix

SURVEY FORM

Name (optional) _____

1. What type of setting (i.e., hospital, school) are you presently working in? _____
   _____

2. In a usual week, how many children between the ages of birth to 12 years do you see?
   (circle one)

   0–5   6–10   11–20   other _____

3. In the past year, how many children maternally exposed to cocaine have you seen?
   (circle one)

   0–3   4–5   6–8   other _____

4. The children maternally exposed to cocaine were seen for: (circle one)

   Treatment   Diagnosis   Both (Tx & Dx)

5. How frequently do you work with the children prenatally exposed to cocaine a week?
   (circle one)

   1–2   3–5   6–7   other _____

6. State the number of children prenatally exposed to cocaine that you see who have as their
   legal guardians:

   HRS _____parents _____

   relative (other than parents) _____other (who?)_____

7. How did you know that the children were reportedly products of a cocaine abuse pregnancy?
   (circle all that apply)

   parent   relative (other than parent)
   family physician   hospital report
   other _____

8. How did you make your original diagnosis of speech and language deficits? (circle one)

   screening   observation   in-depth evaluation

   If the diagnosis was made through an in-depth evaluation, what tests and other protocols
   were used? _____
   _____
   _____

9. Please list deficits found in the following areas by age groups:

birth–2 years	**2.1–4years**
semantics: _____	_____
_____	_____
_____	_____

birth–2 years	**2.1–4 years**

syntax: _____   _____

pragmatics: _____   _____

cognition (i.e., hyperactivity, lack of attention):

_____   _____

physical anomalies: _____   _____

other _____   _____

4.1–6.11 years	**7–older years**

semantics: _____   _____

syntax: _____   _____

pragmatics: _____   _____

cognition (i.e., hyperactivity, lack of attention):

_____   _____

physical anomalies: _____   _____

other: _____   _____